THE RETURN OF THE PLAGUE: BRITISH SOCIETY AND THE CHOLERA 1831–2

Michael Durey

THE RETURN OF THE PLAGUE

British Society and the Cholera 1831-2

GILL AND MACMILLAN
HUMANITIES PRESS

First published in Ireland 1979 by
Gill and Macmillan Ltd
15/17 Eden Quay
Dublin 1
with associated companies in
London, New York, Delhi, Hong Kong,
Johannesburg, Lagos, Melbourne,
Singapore, Tokyo

7171 0970 4

and in the United States of America
by Humanities Press Inc
0–391–01038–7

Printed in Great Britain by
Bristol Typesetting Co. Ltd, Barton Manor, St. Philips, Bristol

Contents

Introduction

EPIDEMICS have long held a particular fascination for both historian and layman alike. One reason for this interest is that histories of past diseases have many of the elements of a good horror story, with whole villages being depopulated, people dropping dead in their tracks, and whole societies nearly grinding to a halt. Another reason for people's curiosity is that epidemics are now only a blur in the folk-memory of Britain, so long is it since this country underwent a severe visitation from a virulent and deadly micro-organism. The history of epidemics thus blends the mysterious, a sense of the unknown or unexperienced, with the exceptional. One of the clearest distinguishing features between the past and the present is the presence of epidemics in the former and their absence in the latter.

Epidemics, however, have a greater function than merely to emphasise the uniqueness of the past; they can also be used as a medium whereby the whole of past societies can be studied, for their arrival always unsettled the normal functioning of society, and brought to the surface latent social antagonisms.

The ways in which society responded to an extraordinary set of circumstances can tell us much about its character which is not easily observable during periods of peace and relative harmony, or at least when underlying social tensions are hidden by the crust of formal social relationships. And if, as in Britain in 1831–2, a new epidemic threat coincided with a period of political crisis, the opportunities for studying the strength and resilience of that society are doubled.

This book investigates the first hesitant responses of British society to the presence of Asiatic or Indian cholera. As its name suggests, cholera was seen by many to be an exotic disease in 1831–2, the period of its first eruption on British soil. Being new, and bringing to an end a long period during which British society was free of any major nationwide epidemic disease, cholera was sure to have repercussions far beyond those associated with endemic diseases such as the fevers, smallpox and tuberculosis. It was, moreover, a disease capable of inducing sheer blind panic, for it struck swiftly and savagely, leaving havoc, pain and distress in its wake.

Into a maelstrom of social, economic and political change in 1831, cholera injected a new and disturbing element, for it tested received attitudes and mentalities, probed society's resources and resourcefulness, and exploited its weaknesses and shortcomings, structural, political, social and moral. Cholera accordingly offers a unique opportunity to study contextually a society under stress, struggling to comprehend and control a new factor in the environment.

Some of the conclusions of this book may surprise. Heavy emphasis is placed on the words *customary, traditional* and *flexible*. Government responses to the disease, as analysed in chapters 1 and 4, were initially traditional, based very much on the lessons which could still be remembered from the time of the plague; indeed, the comparison is startling, if, on reflection, quite understandable. But, when necessary, government agencies could show considerable flexibility, as when Henry Halford's Central Board of Health was dismissed in November 1831, and when government inspectors, usually viewed as a product of Utilitarian planning, were sent into the infected regions. Indeed, the second Central Board of Health came out of the epidemic rather well, even though they accepted their transitory role, and certainly their activities can be compared favourably with the more doctrinaire and rigid system imposed by Edwin Chadwick's Board of Health in 1848–9.

Chapters 2 and 3 are concerned with the relationship between cholera, the environment and socio-economic variables. I attempt to plot the path of cholera through Britain and assess the *local* reasons for the surprisingly low mortality in many of the larger towns, and especially in the manufacturing districts. Equally surprising, people living in non-urban communities in England suffered more, proportionally, than those in the towns. This is explained primarily in terms of local water supplies, the main route by which *V. cholerae* is transmitted. But to get from place to place, cholera travelled in the traditional manner, by foot along the main highways, carried by travellers in what was still a peripatetic society, or by ship around the coast. Chapter 3, a case study of London, uses previously untapped sources to check, at a micro-level, the more general statements made in the previous chapter.

Chapter 4 examines how the national system of local boards of health, established to combat cholera, worked in practice. It is by no means a success story; reliance on such traditional measures as charity, whitewashing and temporary hospitals, collapsed because of popular antipathy to health measures, an antiquated body of health law, and the hesitancy of the central authority facing the need to impose control on the usually autonomous local bodies.

Chapter 5, on medical science and the medical community, rejects the commonly-held view that anti-contagionism became dominant in medical theory around this time. A case is made to suggest that by deliberately relying on traditional remedies, which were neither very successful nor very harmful, the medical profession both did their best for their patients and at the same time improved their status as individual practitioners, although the popularity of the medical community as a whole probably did not increase.

Chapters 6, 7 and 8, the core of the book, deal with mentalities. First, the responses of the propertied classes are examined. The avenues of reaction open to them were wider than for the poor, and conform both to the responses to diseases in previous centuries and to those which have been suggested by present-day psychologists and disaster research theorists. The possible explanations for particular choices of response are examined, and the *chronology* of response is emphasised.

Chapters 7 and 8 are concerned with popular reactions to cholera. All the riots and disturbances in some way connected with the appearance of cholera are examined, and comparisons made between crowd motivations in Britain and Europe. In Britain, no clear evidence of *class* antagonism could be found, although middle-class attempts to forestall cholera sometimes engendered disturbances, while most eruptions were narrowly focused on antagonism towards the medical profession. Chapter 8 deals with the ways in which middle- and working-class leaders incorporated cholera into their world views, and a clear distinction is made between cholera unrest and political and industrial disturbances.

Chapter 9 attempts to draw my themes together, and looks at the impact of cholera during following epidemics. Cholera reaches its peak in 1849 and thereafter declines in virulence as sanitary reform becomes increasingly effective.

For a full understanding of how cholera became a scourge in the nineteenth century and for an explanation of its rapid decline in importance, reference must be made to its specific etiology. Readers who are interested in cholera's particular means of transmission are advised to read the appendix first, where they will find a consideration of those socio-economic variables and environmental conditions which helped or hindered cholera in its journey across Britain.

What emerges from this study, therefore, is a picture of a society which, although undergoing rapid change and at times shaky on its foundations, was basically stable and able to absorb an epidemic with surprising resilience. It thus adds a further dimension to our understanding of how British society withstood, or mediated, the pressures of urbanisation, industrialisation and population growth in the first half of the nineteenth century.

This study is a revised version of my D.Phil thesis, submitted to the University of York in 1975. During its gestation period, I was fortunate enough to be advised and counselled by many friends and colleagues. Peter Tawse kindly drew the maps for me, and Lawrence Hall gave me considerable assistance on the medical aspects of this study. He may not, however, agree with all the conclusions I have drawn from his advice. Others to whom I owe gratitude include James Walvin, John Butcher, Graham Cleator, Margaret Pelling, Ian Inkster and Terry Wyke. I have been fortunate in my typists, my mother for my thesis, Melanie Harris for the final typescript of this study. I thank them both.

Intellectually, I owe much to Gwyn A. Williams, friend, mentor and teacher extraordinary. It was he who first saw the possibilities of some preliminary material on cholera which I had unearthed, and he who, by his constant stimulation and concern, ensured that this study was completed. Those students who have been taught by Gwyn Williams know how fortunate they have been.

But my greatest debt goes to my wife Jill, for translating from the French and Swedish, correcting my grammar and, above all, for showing patience and understanding, even when she found me in the churchyard looking for cholera crosses on our wedding day. To her, and our children, this book is dedicated.

I

Preparations

> We have witnessed in our days the birth of a new pestilence, which in the short space of fourteen years, has desolated the fairest portions of the globe, and swept off at least fifty MILLIONS of our race. It has mastered every variety of climate, surmounted every natural barrier, conquered every people. It has not, like the simoon, blasted life, and then passed away; the cholera, like the smallpox or plague, takes root in the soil it has once possessed.

THUS commented a rather frightened writer in the *Quarterly Review* in November 1831, as cholera first reached the shores of Britain. In fact, cholera was not a new disease, at least not on the Indian sub-continent. The earliest references to a disease which has close similarities to cholera occur in Indian Sanskrit writings of about 400 BC and on a monolith of a temple in Gujrat which dates from the time of Alexander the Great. The inscription on the latter reads, 'the lips blue, the face haggard, the eyes hollow, the stomach sunk in, the limbs contracted and crumpled as if by fire, those are the signs of the great illness which, invoked by a malediction of the priests, comes down to slay the braves'.[1] The tendency of the inhabitants of lower Bengal to worship Oolee Beebe, the goddess of cholera, is testimony to the virulence of the disease in ages past.

But it was not until the nineteenth century that cholera broke out of the Indian sub-continent. After prolonged localised activity from 1769, the first pandemic of cholera began in 1817.[2] Why the disease became of global significance at this time is uncertain, but most probably increased trading links with the rest of the world, combined with abnormal climatic conditions in Bengal between 1815 and 1817, were significant.[3] The original source of the epidemic was Jessore, 'a crowded filthy place, surrounded by marshy and impenetrable jungles'. Cholera's impact was devastating. 'The inhabitants, astonished and terrified at the unaccountable and very destructive inroads of the pestilence, fled in crowds to the country as the only means of escaping impending death.' Within a few weeks, 10,000 were dead.[4] Calcutta was soon infected and at Bundelkand the Marquis of Hastings' army was decimated, 5,000 fatalities occurring before the army broke camp.

After a quiescent period, cholera broke out again in 1818 and engulfed the whole Indian sub-continent. It infected Ceylon and even reached Mauritius in November 1819, 2,000 miles from India, having arrived at the same time as the frigate HMS *Topaze* from Ceylon. By 1824 cholera had covered the whole of South and South-East Asia. Following the northern caravan routes out of India, it had also infected the region of the Caspian, but eventually came to a halt at the gates of Astrakhan in September 1823.

The respite was short-lived, for in 1826 cholera again began its march from Bengal. By August 1829 it had infected Afghanistan, Persia and Orenburg, in the south-east corner of European Russia. From this base cholera, in the spring of 1831, began its journey north-westwards, which was to take it to Moscow, St Petersburg and, in 1831, to Poland and the Baltic ports.[5]

News of cholera's slow but inexorable progress first came to the British government from Lord Haytesbury, British ambassador in St Petersburg, when the disease reached Moscow in September 1830. Haytesbury was not one for minimising the disease's potential danger. 'The accounts published by the government of the ravages of this disease are still sufficiently alarming, but those received by private correspondence are infinitely more so.'[6] Sanitary cordons and quarantine regulations, the principal preventive measures taken by the authorities, had been totally ineffective. They had merely intensified the terror and by 11 September fifty thousand panic-stricken Muscovites were struggling along the roads to St Petersburg and Smolensk.[7] Not even the presence of the tsar could either quell the panic or overawe cholera, which continued to ravage Moscow until the onset of winter reduced its virulence.

The Foreign Office sent Haytesbury's dispatches to the Privy

Council, which at this time was responsible for the nation's rudimentary public health administration. Britain was in fact almost totally unequipped to cope with an invasion of a new and potentially virulent disease. A centralised system of public health did not exist, although both France and Russia possessed central health authorities. In Britain, outside a small group of Benthamites, there was little adherence to the concept of a medical police, i.e., the creation of a medical policy by government and its implementation through administrative regulation. The majority of informed opinion would have been totally opposed to such ideas, for they threatened local autonomy and smacked of the continental sin of centralisation.

The only state medical bodies were the quarantine establishment, the Commission in Lunacy and the Vaccination Board, which were supervised by the Privy Council.[8] Thus, the quarantine system, established to prevent contagious or infectious diseases from entering Britain early in the eighteenth century, was the only means of defence against an epidemic from abroad. Penetration of this curtain by a disease left the country totally unguarded. One can understand this omission as Britain had been free from any widespread infectious epidemic since the last great plague outbreaks in the seventeenth century. This helps to explain why in the first six months of 1831 the Privy Council concentrated on tinkering with its powers under the Quarantine Act. This Act, 6 Geo. IV c .78 (1825), had been the unsuccessful culmination of years of pressure from a group of anticontagionists, whose objective had been the total abolition of the quarantine system.[9] Their activities had backfired and had left the Privy Council with if anything even greater powers and flexibility. Whereas previously exact periods of quarantine were laid down for ships coming from certain ports, the Privy Council could now determine the length of quarantine and could impose it on any ships coming from ports where there were 'alarming or suspicious circumstances as to infection'.

The Privy Council used these powers in November 1830 after the arrival of Haytesbury's dispatches, placing ships arriving in British ports from Russia under a precautionary quarantine, but thereafter nothing was done for several months, although Haytesbury and Sir William Pym, Superintendent General of Quarantine, remained pessimistic.[10] Charles Greville later wrote

'Government was thinking of Reform and other matters and would not bestow much attention upon this subject, and accordingly neither regulations nor preparations were made.'[11] While in justification it is true that cholera remained only a distant threat in the winter of 1830–1, other requirements also precluded government activity. Conflicts of interest severely limited possible courses of action. In particular the Privy Council had to balance the needs of public welfare with the demands of the mercantile and shipowning classes, whose profit margins were at stake. Greville explained the Privy Council's dilemma most neatly.

> The first and most important [responsibility] relates to the conservation of the Public Health, to which every other consideration must undoubtedly give way. But their Lordships are likewise bound to the care that no unnecessary restrictions be imposed upon the trade and commerce of the country; and while on the one hand they will not hesitate to adopt the most rigorous precautions against the introduction of a contagious disease, they cannot determine upon measures calculated most seriously to affect such great various and complicated interests, without the clearest conviction of their unavoidable necessity, and of the danger of the severity of their application.[12]

To sit tight, do nothing and hope that cholera would go away left open the possibility that foreign governments would disrupt British trade by quarantining ships which they could legitimately claim were hazards to health (Britain already had the reputation for being the most inefficient regulator of quarantine in Europe).[13]

Obviously, to defend themselves against criticism, the Privy Council needed some knowledge of the etiology of the disease they faced, but the information they received in the first months of 1831 was conflicting. The essential questions they required answering were: is the disease infectious? and can it, like plague, be transmitted by merchandise? Dr Walker, a St Petersburg physician from whom the Privy Council had sought information, thought the disease to be cholera and not plague, but he declined to judge its possible contagiousness.[14] Accepting at first the non-contagionist ideas then prevalent in Moscow, Walker had returned to St Petersburg along the Volga, being converted to contagionism along the way, although he would not commit himself on the question of goods and merchandise.[15] Thinking he was helping the Privy Council, Walker also sent a report from Dr Albers, an adviser for the Prussian government. Albers unfortunately disagreed with Walker. He too had travelled along the Volga, but in the opposite direction and his views had predictably been altered from contagionism to noncontagionism. He claimed that he had met with 'no instance which could render it at all probable, that the cholera [was] disseminated by inanimate objects'.[16] Other intelligence reaching the Privy Council was equally contradictory and no conclusions could be made, except perhaps, that medical opinions were contagionist in inverse proportion to their distance from the disease.

While the Privy Council vacillated in the spring of 1831, cholera began its onward march and early in May it reached Riga, where between seven and eight hundred British ships were unloading flax and hemp, then regarded as particularly dangerous carriers of the 'contagious principle'.[17] The prospect of cholera arriving within a matter of weeks at one of the northern seaports inspired Sir William Pym to suggest an overhaul of the quarantine system and a call for assistance to the Royal College of Physicians.[18]

The confusion which followed was symptomatic of the chaos and uncertainty which surrounded the whole question of public health at this time. Instead of receiving a judicious medical opinion on the salient problem of the contagiousness of goods, the Privy Council received two contradictory views from the Royal College of Physicians. Sir Henry Halford, President of the College, and three fellows, Thomas Turner, William Macmichael and Francis Bisset Hawkins, swiftly replied that the disease could not be propagated by goods.[19] Later in the week, however, a full meeting of the College rejected this opinion and prudently said that not enough evidence was available for a decision to be made.[20] While the College could claim that the question of quarantine involved more than purely medical considerations and was therefore outside their brief, their position, which they reiterated when Greville gently tried to make them accept Halford's interpretation, again prevented the Privy Council from acting decisively. With clear and unambiguous information still needed, on 17 June the Privy Council dispatched Doctors Russell and Barry, both of whom had experience of cholera, to Riga.[21]

While they waited for the reports, the Privy Council considered possible second lines of defence against cholera. Their first inclination was to look backwards in time for inspiration. The Council found that precedents existed in emergencies for an official General (or Central) Board of Health. Richard Mead had suggested one during a plague scare in 1721 and a Central Board had been established in 1805 when it was feared yellow fever would reach Britain.[22] The Privy Council followed the pattern of 1805 and on 18 June established a board of health of eleven men, six representing the medical profession and five various government and military departments.[23] It is worth considering in some detail the composition of this board, because from it the Privy Council expected to obtain the medical and administrative expertise necessary to combat cholera. On the medical side the board was heavily weighted in favour of the elitist Royal College of Physicians. Sir Henry Halford was president of the board and he chose the other five medical members. His selection added fuel to the fires of controversy concerning the Fellows' monopoly of the plums of the profession and ensured that the less prestigious branches of the profession and the radical press would regard the board with disfavour. By 1830 the Royal College of Physicians was out of touch with modern scientific developments. It still saw the physician's role as that of a gentleman, and its hierarchical structure ensured that natural talent failed to gain its just reward. Halford epitomised the College's glittering but hollow image. One of the five eminent sons of Dr James Vaughan, he had gradually emerged as the most exclusive doctor in London, becoming Physician Extraordinary to four successive monarchs. Although earning about £10,000 a year, he was by no means an exceptional physician. While he had obviously cultivated the bedside manner to a fine art, he did not believe it necessary physically to examine his patients, nor was he experienced in pathology.[24]

Of the five other physicians on the board, only Pelham Warren's medical reputation exceeded his social standing.[25] William Macmichael, Halford's right hand man, had just become Physician in Ordinary to William IV (at Halford's instigation). His reputation rested more on his authorship of *The Gold Headed Cane*, a work on the lives of the Presidents of the Royal College, than on any medical attainments.[26] William Maton was more interested in botany than medicine and his books did not show 'much depth of medical attainment'. Perhaps predictably, only Halford had a larger practice in London. Thomas Turner was Treasurer of the Royal College and Sir Henry Holland preferred the delights of travel and society to the more mundane life of a hospital physician. He settled for earning £5,000 a year and 'knew everybody'.[27]

Social prestige played a smaller part in the appointment of the five administrators to the board. Pym was a natural choice. His contagionist beliefs were grounded on years of personal experience of infectious diseases. Although he had no experience of cholera, Pym had unrivalled knowledge of yellow fever. He had been in the West Indies during the epidemic of 1794–6 and had in 1815 published *Observations upon Bulam Fever* which asserted, against much contemporary opinion, yellow fever's contagiousness. Pym's appointment as Superintendent General of Quarantine in 1826 should be seen as a deliberate provocation to that small group of liberal noncontagionist medical men who had sought quarantine's abolition.[28]

Practical experience of health administration was gained by the appointment of Sir James McGrigor and Sir William Burnett. McGrigor had served throughout the world (including India and Egypt) during the Napoleonic Wars and in 1815 had been appointed Director General of the Army Medical Board. This was renowned for its corruption and exclusive patronage, but he had completely remodelled it and initiated the system of army medical reports, the statistics from which he used, twenty years before Edwin Chadwick and William Farr thought of it, to establish regulations for the preservation of the health of the troops. Sir William Burnett was Physician General to the Navy, where he had carried out similar reforms to McGrigor's, ordering ships' surgeons to make periodic, nosologically arranged returns for each hospital and ship. He had also given his support to the naval assistant surgeons in their campaign for better conditions. The final appointment to the board was Admiral Sir Thomas Byam Martin, Comptroller of the Navy and government placeman in parliament. He was a sound administrator and had experience of Riga, having taken part in its defence against Marshal Davout in 1812.[29]

The board of health was, therefore, composed of two different interest groups. On the one hand were the physicians, all Fellows of the Royal College and all, except Holland, products of Oxford and Cambridge. Ignorant of cholera, redolent of social success and prestige, they had few real medical attributes. Halford was to blame for their presence on the board. Admittedly the Privy Council had asked him to choose his colleagues, but it is difficult to see what the alternatives were. Thomas Wakley, editor of the radical medical journal *The Lancet*, disagreed and accused the Privy Council of trafficking in patronage.

> Emanating from the Privy Council, with Majesty at its head, Sir Henry Halford of course stands prominent; for wherever there is the face of royalty we are sure to find the nose of Sir Henry Halford . . . He may be well qualified to instruct us how to endure the noxious atmosphere of a Court; but God protect us from the infliction of his conservative measures . . . The appointment of such a person is a scandal to the profession, an insult to those able practitioners who have served in India, and a mockery to the alarmed feelings of the public.[30]

Yet without an established public health department, the Privy Council could turn to no other institution. There were certainly East India Company surgeons in Britain who had treated cholera patients, but in June 1831 the Privy Council did not know for sure that the disease in the Baltic was cholera. Following tradition, the Council had to appoint Halford and they could hardly then refuse his nominations. They did the next best thing, therefore, and balanced the board by their own five appointments. They set against the inherent conservatism and social prestige of the Royal College of Physicians the moderate liberalism, flexibility and proven talent of men like McGrigor and Burnett (the former, as so many of his generation, had embraced Jacobin ideas for a time when a student); the healing art of the physicians was balanced by the more pragmatic surgical and administrative experience of the military men; and the experience of drawing-room illness was counteracted by the experience of infectious diseases, although no one on the board had any first-hand knowledge of cholera.

In only one way was the Board's composition distorted; a majority of the members believed in the theories of contagionism. Prudence dictated that the board should be weighted in that way, for in June 1831 no concrete evidence existed to support any alternative hypothesis. But there were degrees of contagionism, stretching from contingent contagionism, where an atmospheric or localised poison could in certain circumstances be transmitted from person to person, to the extreme position where goods and merchandise, as well as people, could act as vectors. Given the obligations to trading interests, the closer to contingent contagionism the board of health could come, the happier the Privy Council would be. The duties of the board of health, to suggest modifications to the quarantine system, to decide on the question of goods as vectors and to prepare regulations to prevent 'cholera's *contagious* spread' if it did arrive, all point to the Privy Council's refusal to countenance noncontagionist or miasmatic ideas.[31]

The Royal College of Physicians' refusal to move from the extreme position on 18 June was confirmed by the board of health's similar refusal on 22 June. Indeed, the board suggested strengthening the machinery of the quarantine service. This was done, although Greville complained that 'All evidence proves that goods are not capable of bringing the disorder, but we have appointed a Board of Health, which is contagionist, and we can't get them to subscribe to that opinion. . . . So we are obliged to air goods. . . . We have gone on pretty well hitherto, but more ships arrive every day.'[32] On the Medway, the failure to construct a permanent quarantine site during the previous fifty years left the Admiralty with no choice but to use Sheerness as a quarantine station, a ludicrous situation for it put the town's ten thousand population at immediate risk. John Hearncorn, a local surgeon, warned that the infection would inevitably move from Sheerness to London 'when we shall have all the dismal scenes of 1665 renewed'.[33] Fortunately the quarantine regulations were rigorously enforced and although cholera broke out on some ships from Riga at Standgate Creek (the quarantine station off Sheerness), the disease did not spread to the shore.[34]

The Privy Council's dissatisfaction with the board of health was heightened by the proposed regulations, submitted on 28 June and 11 July, to deal with cholera if it did arrive. They had originated from a subcommittee consisting of Sir Willam Burnett and Drs Warren and Macmichael, all of whom were avowed contagionists. The regulations proposed that as soon as cholera was confirmed in a town, 'expurgators' should take the victims on special conveyances to a temporary lazaretto ('pest-house'). Those who had been in contact with the sick should likewise be taken to another house, preferably close to the lazaretto so they could be transferred if necessary. 'In this removal Police Officers or Military should be on duty to prevent any approach to the expurgators, the sick, or the suspected, or to carriages in which the sick are conveyed to the lazarettos.'[35] No one should be allowed contact with the sick or suspected, unless they were prepared to accept the same regimen. The dead should be buried as close to the lazaretto as possible. The regulations ended,

> The Board are fully aware of the aggravation of individual misery consequent on the separation of members of the same family, but private feelings must give way to the public safety, and the state has a right to expect from its subjects an acquiescence in means of indispensable General Policy.

The shadow of the Great Plague hangs heavily over these proposals. They were 'formed to meet a case of virulent infection equalled only by the plague in its fatal consequences'. The Board certainly made use of old plague treatises before they drew up their proposals.[36] But to conflate cholera with plague, which most people accepted was one of the most contagious diseases known to man, filled the Privy Council with horror. Both rural and urban areas were at this time in a state of acute discontent. The abnormally high price of cereals, the introduction of labour-saving agricultural machinery and the influence of the July revolution in France had led to serious disturbances in the agricultural South and Midlands at the end of 1830. By June 1831 agitation for the Reform Bill was growing. Already one Bill had been lost in March 1831, and rioting had occurred in the subsequent elections. Now, only a few days before the Board had sent in its report, the Reform Bill had passed its second reading in the House of Commons. In that same month troops were used to quell riots in Merthyr, in which more than twenty civilians were killed. The police force, at work only in metropolitan London, was equally unpopular. Most Englishmen were convinced that the use of troops and police undermined their traditional birthright of personal freedom from arbitrary authority.[37] It was impossible for the Privy Council to accept regulations which might have resulted in troops being sent into working-class areas. Confrontation between the people and the forces of law and order was the last thing they wanted. Nor would sanitary cordons around infected areas have been possible. 'If strictly enforced', warned John Marshall of Port Glasgow, 'it would shake the whole fabric of society to its very basis, excite the most serious discontent and end as in Russia by being totally futile in arresting the progress of the malady.'[38]

The Lords of the Privy Council were hamstrung by their own board of health. Acting, thought Greville, under the ultra-contagionist and safety-conscious influence of Dr Warren, the board had totally failed to appreciate the wider view of affairs which the Privy Council had to take. Yet their lordships could not reject the regulations outright. The board of health had been established purely as an advisory body, but in practice it had some power. The Council could not be seen rejecting opinions which might in the future guarantee public health. As Greville noted, 'We dare not act without [the board's] sanction.'[39]

The only alternative was to do nothing, but as professional medical bodies increasingly sought information and as the board of health pressed for a firm decision, the Privy Council permitted some of the less objectionable regulations to be issued to those who requested them. But the rules were to be available only to professional bodies until cholera was officially declared present in Britain—hardly the best way of using them to advantage, for they were largely concerned with preventing cholera from arriving at all.

Rumours that sanitary cordons would be part of government policy quickly circulated. Wakley wrote caustically in *The Lancet*, 'Sagacious legislators, who cannot prevent the cholera from traversing the ocean, yet can keep it from penetrating a hedge, or crossing a field.'[40] All the evidence from abroad demonstrates that government attempts to conquer cholera by throwing military picket lines around infected areas would be not only naïve but also dangerous. In the whole of Eastern Europe coercive measures produced a common response, a deep unrest among the poor culminating in riots and murder. The major lesson the Privy Council learned in these months was that central government intervention was counterproductive. The European poor regarded attempts to help them as an exercise in mass murder. Russell and Barry first reported this phenomenon from St Petersburg. All foreigners and medical men, they said, were regarded with suspicion. They personally were unable to help during the epidemic because the poor thought they had come to poison them. Already in June one German physician had been murdered and six others severely beaten. Russell and Barry seemed to believe the conspiracy theory.

> It is certain that individuals have been apprehended here since the commencement of the epidemic, with poisonous substances of considerable quantity, such as corrosive sublimate, and arsenic about their persons and, though poorly dressed, carrying large sums of money. Two such persons were put to death by the mob, and others are in custody. It would appear that the popular mind had been worked up by these circumstances into a belief that the cholera morbus owed its origins to these emissaries.[41]

The riots spread to the Russian military colonies, where peasants massacred physicians and magistrates who had been employed to enforce the sanitary cordons.[42]

When cholera spread into Prussia the lowest classes refused to believe that a new disease existed. Cholera deaths were ascribed to poison administered by doctors, bribed to kill off the surplus population, an ingenious method supposedly already used effectively by the British in India. 'The foreign doctors who have been sent to Russia, Poland and Prussia to observe the disease are according to this hypothesis the delegates of a central committee consisting of a hundred members formed in London and who direct the whole proceedings.'[43] The Prussian king, it was claimed, was paying doctors between two and three thalers for every death they caused. Such ideas circulated in all the country areas and also in some of the towns.

The same scenario was played out in the Austrian Empire. Burdensome regulations caused political tumult and the appearance of the poison theory. In Hungary the disease was particularly deadly, over one hundred thousand dying between June and September 1831. 'The populace, finding themselves thus exposed to an enemy who made what appeared to them so invidious a distinction between the rich and the poor . . . took up the idea that the pretended disease was a conspiracy of the upper classes to sweep away by poison their miserable inferiors.' Peasants sacked castles and murdered noblemen, quarantine officers and doctors. Poison (actually chlorate of lime) was discovered in the cellars of castles, thus confirming the rumours.[44]

If the ends had justified the means there might have been some point in government intervention. But all the evidence pointed to its futility, and every East European state eventually came to the same conclusion. In Prussia the sanitary cordons were withdrawn before cholera reached Berlin, and in Vienna the Emperor admitted that cordons and quarantine had produced 'consequences more mischievous than those resulting from the malady itself'.[45] The Russian government abandoned quarantine in August 1831 once the whole country was infected, although the tsar kept a double sanitary cordon around Peterhof.[46]

The East European states gave up their preventive measures at the very time when the Privy Council had to decide whether to implement the board of health's regulations and when the French Chamber of Deputies had just voted one million francs for sanitary cordons.[47] Greville believed the stories coming from Europe were nonsense, but he could not afford to ignore them. In *The Lancet* a writer calling himself *Alpha* warned that the effect of quarantine and cordons was 'to increase [the disease's] ravages a hundredfold, to ruin the country, and to make the people revolt against measures which draw down on them misery and death at the same time'.[48] There was no reason why this reaction should not come as easily from a downtrodden and discontented English workforce as from European peasants. Greville saw this as further confirmation of the futility of the board of health's recommendations. Throughout August and September the Privy Council was receiving information from Europe, much of which strengthened their hand against the board of health. Russell and Barry were certain that what they were witnessing was not plague but a disease new to Europe; it appeared to be contagious from man to man but not from goods.[49] Dr Hamett, a physician from Danzig, sent four reports to London (the first of which seems to have been suppressed by the board of health),[50] in which he tried to prove that cholera was not contagious at all.

The Privy Council had to act at the beginning of October when the cholera reached Hamburg, only a three-day journey by steamship from Britain. Almost certainly the board of health was pressured into submitting less controversial proposals, which were ready by 12 October. No mention was made of forcible removal. Just how forceful the Privy Council had been we do not know, nor do we know whether some members of the board were more ready to concede ground than others. The two pieces of evidence extant are a letter from William Macmichael to his fellow board members dated 6 October and a revised copy of the rules and regulations. Macmichael had expunged all the 'frightful words' such as expurgators and lazarettos from the document. He admitted to remaining faithful to the board's original position, but at the same time he injected some badly needed realism into the discussion.

> Until the government can get the public to co-operate with them, for a conviction of the reasonableness of these measures, no good will ever be done. As to the isolation of particular districts, it is an affair of military police, and may be made more or less strict, according to the power and authority of the government to enforce it. But the question is, what are the unfortunate people to do, in whose district the disease may appear? Are you to wall them up, allow them to perish and only take care that the pestilence does not spread further than that detested spot?

The rules should be published, 'for surely though a great part of our free countrymen may choose to die like rotten sheep in their own way, yet the well-disposed and sober-minded ought to know what measures may protect them.'[51]

The resultant proposals accepted by the Privy Council were a compromise. The sick were to go to temporary hospitals only if they or their relatives agreed. If they refused, families suffering from cholera were to remain in isolation in their own homes, with the word SICK emblazoned on their doors, until the period of convalescence was completed. Infected houses were to be thoroughly cleansed and the dead buried in a detached plot of ground. No mention was made of sanitary cordons, although local magistrates should attempt 'by the best means in their power' to prevent communication with an infected town. The final warning allowed board members to save face.

> Other measures, of a more coercive nature, may be rendered expedient for a common safety, if unfortunately so fatal a disease should ever show itself in this country in the terrific way in which it has appeared in various parts of Europe; and it may become necessary to draw troops, or a strong body of police, around infected places, so as utterly to exclude the inhabitants from all intercourse with the country.[52]

There is no doubt that the government was heavily influenced by the evidence of disturbances abroad. The regulations were altered 'in consequence of the violent opposition raised in various capitals in Europe, to all attempts made to enforce more rigid regulations'.[53] Fear of rioting, if not of revolution, forced the Privy Council's hand, and as Pym later admitted to his French counterpart, Moreau de Jonnès, 'In this country, we cannot establish a cordon by land . . . from the apprehension of the same results as occurred in St Petersburg, Hungary and other places.'[54] In Britain, the political situation had worsened dramatically since June. On 8 October the second Reform Bill had been defeated in the House of Lords, partly because of episcopal opposition. The immediate consequence was rioting in Worcester, Bath, Derby and Nottingham culminating in the sacking of Bristol at the end of October. As one historian has noted, 'Viewed from one aspect, England was without any doubt passing through a crisis . . . in which revolution was possible.'[55]

The Order in Council establishing the new regulations was published on 20 October. The real irony had become apparent the day before when the Attorney General reported that the powers given to the Privy Council by the 1825 Quarantine Act were insufficient to make the regulations obligatory.[56] All the Privy Council could do was suggest that they be carried out. After all the discussion between the Council and the board of health, the compromise regulations could not be enforced, even when the disease had reached Britain. All hopes of a central body overseeing a coherent preventive policy now depended on the good sense of the ruling classes in every town and parish. Fortunately, the board of health, with its one flash of real originality, had proposed that each parish in the country should establish a local board of health, on which local interests, the magistracy, the clergy, the medical profession and the ruling elites, were to be represented. The local boards, although some were to function only spasmodically and with little enthusiasm, were harnessed in defence of the public's health.

If this recommendation was, in the future, to save the reputation of the government, in the short term the Order in Council had a poor reception. Unaware that it was a compromise and that fiercer regulations had been shelved, objections were raised on many grounds. The invidious threat of central intervention was explicit; the Order still smacked of the seventeenth-century plague regulations; public health measures should be the responsibility of the local medical men and no one else; and a powerful system of medical police should have been established.[57] The most comprehensive attack on the Privy Council's proposals came from the tory *Quarterly Review*. In the November edition Robert Ferguson, a distinguished obstetrician and man of letters, posed a series of questions which he believed the board of health had manifestly failed to answer.

> Have the king's ministers endeavoured to bring home to their own minds the effects of a sudden paralysation of commerce through every limb of our body politic? Have they tried to calculate the consequences of prodigious masses of artisans—and in times like these too—being sunk at once to the depths of pauperism? Have they considered the necessity of guarding us, in case of the evil coming upon in its most frightful form against the rapacity of monopolists as respects goods and fuel? Have they begun to think of public stores of bread? . . . Have they begun to make arrangements as to hospitals? Have they warned our medical officers, naval and military, that their services may be called for at a moment's notice? Have they considered what ought to be done as to the supply of our markets—the supply of medicine and medical skill to a population dislocated in all its joints, and stricken in all its resources—the regulations as to travellers, inns and public conveyances of all kinds? Have they even dreamed of the enormous burden of care that may within a week devolve on them as a cabinet?[58]

Ferguson was panic-stricken and fearful for the safety of his class. Would a member of any class other than the middle have suggested that all superfluous domestics should be got rid of, and that 'all vagabonds, beggars and old-clothesmen must disappear'? The spectre of the working class haunted his vision.

> Every historian of pestilence, from Thucydides to Jonnès, abounds in awful descriptions of the outbursts of crime that inevitably attends such visitations; and as it is obvious that this can only proceed from the suspension of usual occupations, it is needful to enquire what occupations are the most sure to be interrupted—and what nation can ever have had such reasons to fear, in respect of such a calamity, as the one that possesses the most enormous proportion of manufacturers (*sic*) that the world has ever witnessed?

Only strong government action, he felt, could prevent disaster. 'The more rigorous the laws and the more strictly they are enforced, the more certainly will the government be pronounced a merciful one, at the time by the intelligent, in the sequel by all.'

Ferguson reflected the fears of many at this time, but he was being less than fair to the board of health, for many of the questions he had posed had already been considered. The board had been in touch with the London hospitals and had asked the Privy Council in June for several medical men with experience of cholera to be chosen to help at short notice. Sir James McGrigor informed all the half-pay army medical men that their services might be required. Experiments (which failed) were carried out to discover if chlorine was an effective disinfecting agent and some attempt was made to examine the state of some of the London streets.[59] Within their limited jurisdiction, therefore, the board did take some hesitant steps towards answering many of Ferguson's questions. But they had no mandate to consider the greater questions of social policy nor, in fairness, would they probably have been capable of dealing with them if they had had the opportunity. They at least had been prepared to countenance strong government action if the disease had reached Britain.

Such press criticisms could be withstood. What brought down the board of health was criticism which accentuated the policy split between the board and its parent body. Knowing Greville's low opinion of the members of the board of health (and Greville probably represented official Privy Council policy), any attack on the composition of the board was likely to be effective. For instance, Halford's employment of his own cronies was unpopular. 'Instead of labouring to produce a sound, sightly, well-constructed "board", [Halford] appears to have kept his eye upon inert worthless blocks; or as a correspondent aptly expresses it, "Sir Henry could fix upon none but his own intimate friends and toadies".'[60] Immediately, the board became the target for all those who aimed at the discomfiture of the Royal College of Physicians. Pym was attacked for being contagionist in order to make money, although there is no evidence that Pym deliberately 'puffed' contagionism as a means of personal profit. *Alpha*'s opinion that Pym 'enjoys his good quarantine pay, his good half pay from another department . . . and . . . a smart pension of which only a few are aware' may have been true, but there is no doubt that he honestly believed in contagionism and had said so for many years before he became Superintendent General of Quarantine.[61] Nor was it true that each member of the board would receive £500 per annum for their services.[62] For their five months' work each received £125, not a large amount when compared with Halford's average earnings. Their total expenses came to £76.[63]

The critics were on stronger ground when they condemned the board's stubbornness. Certainly the board was obdurate in its refusal to consider the possibility that cholera was not contagious. It was widely believed at the time that most of the East India Company surgeons were noncontagionists, but the board only bothered to interview seven, although according to their own records eighty-four retired Indian medical officers were then living in Britain and more than a hundred were on furlough at the beginning of 1832.[64] Only one of the seven avowed the non-contagionist philosophy and another four failed to commit themselves. Obviously the board did not go out of its way to hear both sides of the argument.

What really undermined the credibility of the board was its ability to antagonise everyone, not just the noncontagionists (who tended to be the 'progressives' and therefore had two reasons for opposing the board), but also the uncommitted or undecided. The whiff of corruption surrounding the board was unpleasant, as was Halford's oracular manner. The board was too unbending and, though Halford had said in June that the board would be amenable to new evidence, later that month he had publicly supported Macmichael's newly published pamphlet defending contagionism.[65] Macmichael refuted the notion that contagionism was an old prejudice whose only purpose was to act as a chopping block for the 'liberal spirit of enquiry of the present day'.[66] Here was the nub of the board's unpopularity. Halford was the 'Eldon' of his profession, a medical backwoodsman, and the board of health was compared with the reactionary House of Lords. Contagionism, with its natural partner quarantine, did not reflect the spirit of the age. *Alpha* had hinted at this when he observed that Halford's view of cholera was unimportant 'at this time of reform in everything'. The Privy Council was not pleased with being tarred by the same brush, taking responsibility for decisions with which they did not wholeheartedly agree.

It only needed proof that cholera had reached this country for the board of health to be quietly replaced. Isolated cases had occurred in Sunderland in August, but the main epidemic began towards the end of October, with a spate of cases which confirmed suspicions that Sunderland had the least effective quarantine system in Britain. The reports of the government inspector Robert Daun from Sunderland in the first week of November, confirming the existence of Asiatic cholera, sealed the fate of Halford's board of health.

On 12 November the board learned that a new Central Board of Health had been established at the Privy Council office. The physicians on Halford's board were invited to continue as an advisory body, although Greville noted in his diary that it was intended to make the old board 'a mere nullity'. It continued to meet occasionally and was even asked whether the quarantine regulations should be relaxed. Halford replied that nothing in the new evidence persuaded him to change his mind. The old board went down with its colours tied to the mast. It had not been a total failure, for quarantine, without doubt, worked for a while; the number of cases of cholera on ships undergoing purification testified to that. Obviously, in an age when the germ theory was unknown, quarantine could not have kept infectious diseases at bay indefinitely, but when used efficiently it was certainly preferable to the fatalism or false confidence of the noncontagionists.

The board may have been jobbers, they may have been naïve and biased, but it is arguable that quarantine regulations kept cholera out of Britain at least until the dangerous months for the disease's spread (August and September) had slipped by.

2

The Diffusion of Cholera through Britain

THE comparatively late arrival of cholera in Sunderland in October 1831 prevented the disease from spreading very rapidly throughout the town, for the cooler weather inhibited its progress. However, between October 1831 and the end of February 1832 cholera spread from Sunderland to infect nearly the whole of North-East England.[1] Most at risk were the inhabitants of Newcastle, which was officially declared infected on 27 November, but the diffusion of cholera was in all directions: south-west to Penshaw and Houghton-le-Spring by 1 December; south to Seaham harbour and north to Sedghill colliery by the 10th; and south-east along the Tyne to North Shields, also by the 10th.[2] The disease was soon spreading indiscriminately, infecting Gateshead, Wallsend, Morpeth, Byton, Newburn, Durham, Stockton, Jarrow and the colliery villages at Walker, Percy Main, Earsdon and Backworth. Once Newcastle had been infected, it acted as the hub from which cholera radiated throughout the North-East. In particular, cholera struck villages along the Tyne and many of the colliery villages which dotted the Northumberland and Durham landscape. Although cholera's progress was slow, the unusually mild weather in the late autumn enabled the disease to keep a firm grip on the North-East.[3] By February 1832 most of the Tyne region was infected: cholera had reached every hamlet on the north bank from Newburn to North Shields, and to the south it had penetrated an area two miles either side of Gateshead.

The failure to impose sanitary cordons or to restrict trade from infected areas enabled cholera to break out of the North-East by the New Year. An isolated case of cholera had been reported in a Lancaster workhouse on 17 December 1831, but it was the outbreak at Haddington on Christmas Day which signalled cholera's advance, for it was around this small town, only eighteen miles from Edinburgh on the main mail coach route from London, that cholera took a firm hold. Reaching Edinburgh by 22 January, cholera marched slowly westwards until by the end of March the whole of the Scottish lowlands, including Glasgow and Paisley, were infected.

The disease, however, took longer to spread southwards into England. Apart from isolated cases in Knaresborough and Doncaster, no new focal point existed until London became infected in February. Strong trading links between the coal producing North-East and the capital had always made a direct infection of London likely. The doubtful honour of attending the first suspected case in London fell to Mr Bowie, a surgeon practising in the East Smithfield area, who fifteen years later was to play a prominent role as Edwin Chadwick's principal witness at the Metropolitan Sanitary Commission enquiry. On 7 February Bowie informed the Central Board of Health of the death of one Daniel Barber, a sailor from the *Felicity* out of Limerick. Barber had been seen in a 'state of collapse, blue, cold and pulseless and suffering severely from spasms'.[4] Because the victim had been in London for three weeks and had not arrived from the North-East, the Central Board refused to accept the case as genuine, although they took the precaution of ordering the *Felicity* to Standgate Creek quarantine station.

Their respite was short-lived, for within a week eleven cases of cholera had occurred in London. The first was that of 48 year-old John James on 8 February, who died within eight hours of the doctor visiting his home in Hanover Street, Rotherhithe. He had been a shipscraper on the Regent's Canal and on the day of his illness had been working on the *Elizabeth*, a collier from Newcastle. The Central Board accepted James as the first official case in the capital, but he had been predeceased by a 62 year-old labourer from Mint Street, Southwark. Florance Sullivan, 'previously reputed to be a strong and healthy man' though subject to bowel disorders, contracted the disease in the early hours of 8 February after consuming a supper of sprats. Within seventeen hours he was dead.[5]

John James had almost certainly become infected while at work. The southern end of the Regent's Canal stretches through the parish of St Anne, Limehouse, and here the next fatalities occurred, those of Margaret Shea, her daughter Caroline and Mary Ferguson, a woman of 'loose character'. On the Sunday that Ferguson died Mrs Roberts of Bear Garden, Southwark, took a stroll with her husband. Returning home she fell ill and swiftly succumbed to all the dreadful symptoms of the new disease. 'Of spare habit and addicted to dram drinking', she died that same night.[6] Together with a coaldredger and an unemployed sailor in Rotherhithe, a child in Mrs Roberts' house and two sailors on the river, these were the first cases of cholera in London.[7]

By 20 February seven parishes had become infected, forty cases and twenty-one deaths having been reported. From the two original foci of Southwark and Limehouse the disease spread slowly along the Thames. Whitechapel, where many sailors, coal-heavers and other river workers lived, was the first parish not bordering the river to become infected, and by the 25th, Marylebone, St Pancras, St Giles and Bermondsey had reported cases.[8]

This first phase of the epidemic in London demonstrated the effect cool weather had in hindering cholera's progress, for a month passed before most of the parishes had reported cases; by the middle of April the Central Board of Health believed that the disease was waning sufficiently for eight of the twelve medical inspectors in the capital to be given three weeks notice.[9] By 8 May London was declared free of cholera, having escaped relatively lightly. Southwark alone, with 859 cases and 420 deaths, suffered one-third of the casualties, although only one-twentieth of the population lived there. Both Newington and Bermondsey suffered considerably, but north of the Thames only St Giles and Marylebone were badly affected (in absolute terms).[10]

Table 2.1 shows that the Central Board was right to believe in cholera's decline in May, but the disease continued to smoulder in pockets both sides of the Thames. Between 7 May and 15 June cases were reported from Westminster, the Strand, the City, Limehouse and Newington. From about 26 May cholera began to spread again, the new focal point being the eastern working-class parishes. The London newspapers, at first unaware of cholera's recrudescence, began to report new cases only at the beginning of July, as the whole of London became infected. This second

Table 2.1 : Monthly Cholera Morbidity and Mortality in London, 1832

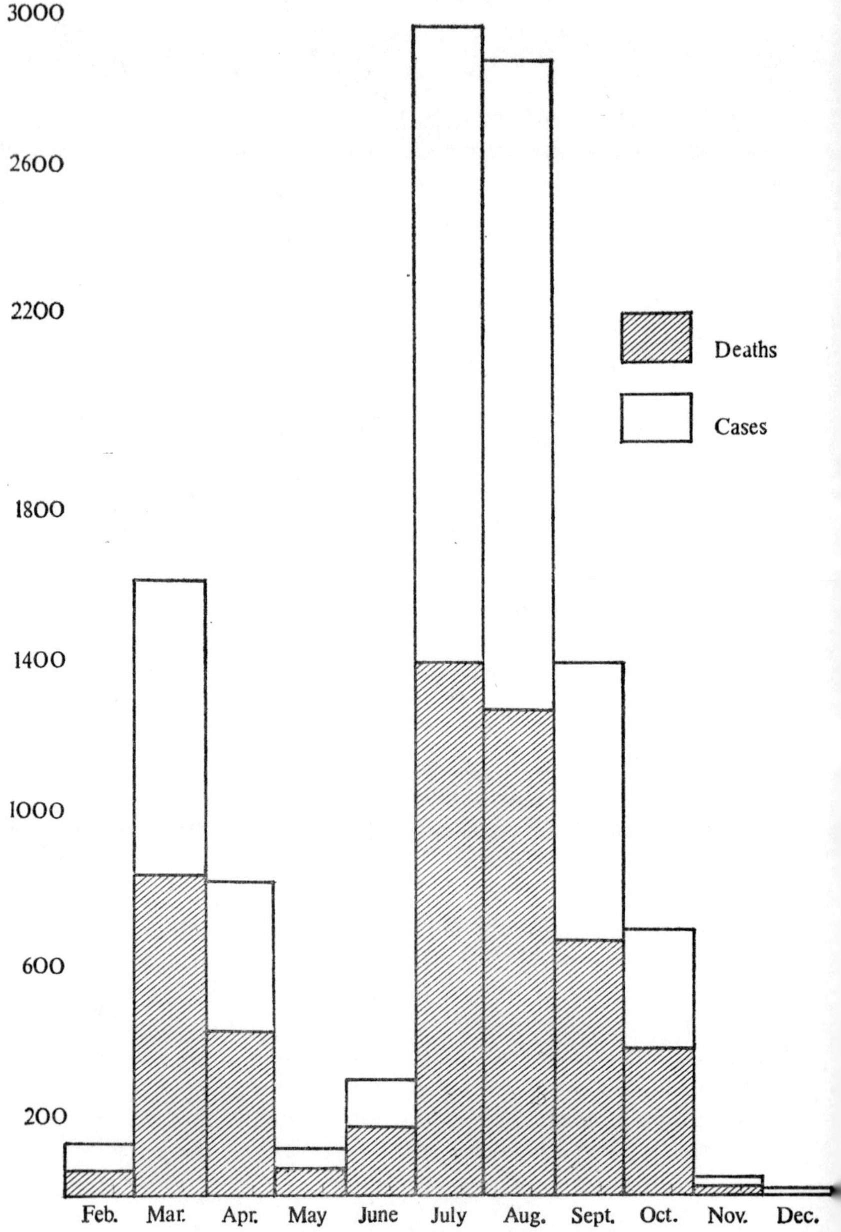

Source: Barry, 'On the Statistics of Cholera', 88.

upsurge was to be much more virulent than the first. Those parishes infected before May had gained no immunity, but in the second outbreak *every* parish suffered, including the outlying parishes such as Hackney and Fulham. Both phases of the epidemic lasted about a hundred days, but from the end of September the disease began to disappear from those inner parishes which had been the first re-infected in June. It was primarily the out-parishes, from a line through Clerkenwell, Old Street and Bethnal Green, north and eastwards, where cholera remained into November. The last parish to report the disease's disappearance was All Saints', Poplar, on 15 November. The official returns for the period 15 June to December 1832 put the number of cases in London at 9,172 and the deaths at 4,281.[11]

While cholera was spreading slowly through London in the spring, only a few other areas of England were infected. Until the end of March cholera kept fairly close to the eastern seaboard, but isolated cases occurred in Dudley and Worcester. In April cholera began to spread inland, following the Humber estuary and the Yorkshire Ouse through Goole, Selby, Hull and Market Weighton. It was in June, however, that cholera took its first major strides which led to its dispersion over wide tracts of Britain. It spread along the Aire and Calder Navigation to Leeds, broke out in Liverpool and infected parts of North Wales and Oxfordshire. Twenty-eight towns and villages reported the presence of cholera in May (see Table 2.2). No longer did the

Table 2.2: New Cholera Outbreaks in Britain, October 1831 to December 1832

1831	October	1	1832	May	28
	November	1		June	59
	December	13		July	75
				August	79
1832	January	20		September	63
	February	12		October	41
	March	20		November	8
	April	26		December	1

Sources: Cholera Returns of Great Britain, PC1/108; Mins. of C.Bd, PC1/105.

disease keep fairly consistently to the periphery of eastern England, only infecting towns either close to the coast or on the estuaries of major rivers. Coinciding with the warmer weather cholera spread westwards at an increasingly rapid pace. Nottingham, Manchester and Plymouth became new focal points of the disease and it took a firm grip on Yorkshire, Lancashire, Oxfordshire, Lincolnshire and Kent. In June fifty-nine new outbreaks were reported, more than twice the number for May.

The peak of the epidemic came with the summer months of July, August and September, when the boards of health of 217 towns and villages sent reports to London. In these months the industrial regions of Staffordshire, Warwickshire and Shropshire suffered very severely, as did the South-West when cholera spread from Plymouth, Bristol and Exeter. Wales was largely spared, but in Scotland the disease traversed the lowlands again and worked its way up the eastern coastal area of the Highlands. At the height of the epidemic few counties were entirely free of cholera, although some purely rural regions such as Sussex, Wiltshire and Herefordshire remained healthy.

With the return of cooler weather in October cholera's hold began to slacken and by November the epidemic was virtually over. A small outbreak in Knaresborough in December proved to be the last reported to the Central Board. Cholera was to return in 1833, to London as well as to some rather unexpected places, but its passage was virtually unnoticed.[12]

The study of cholera's diffusion during this first epidemic confirms the opinion of modern epidemiologists that 'the pathways of infection correspond to the systems of human communications made in proportion to their relative frequency and permeability. . . . The contributing factors are essentially human contacts.'[13] The rapidity and extent of cholera's diffusion, therefore, was constrained partly by the limitations of the transportation network. Coastal shipping was to be important in carrying cholera over long distances to new focal points, but it was the means of human communications within Britain, the turnpike and canal systems, which enabled the disease to penetrate the hinterland. No official restrictions were placed on the internal communications network in 1832. Half-thought out and half-implemented ideas on disease restriction resulted in the anomalous situation whereby all internal traffic was free to proceed as usual from infected parts of Britain. As one Sheffield newspaper noted, cholera 'is welcomed to the Metropolis in a chaise and pair, or even a stage waggon, by any of the great northern roads—but, under sundry pains and penalties, he must not come in a coal barge up the Thames'.[14] The value of quarantine regulations for coastal shipping was demonstrated by the failure of cholera to spread from the North-East down the coast during the winter of 1831–2. But once the disease struck London and the warmer weather arrived, the major seaports around the English coast slowly became infected. There seems little doubt that the cause of their infection was the arrival of ships from already unhealthy ports.

These ports in turn became foci for the disease, even though they were hundreds of miles from the major infected areas. Cholera then extended inland from the ports by means of travellers. The overland carriage of disease was the major means whereby cholera was diffused throughout Britain in 1832. This applied even during the colder months early in the epidemic. Haddington certainly became infected by the overland route, although this was denied at the time. There were two possible sources of infection, one being a group of cobblers who had left Newcastle on foot on 14 December, reaching Haddington five days later. However, the first case, a very dissipated individual who had slept outdoors in a drunken stupor the night before, occurred in Haddington before the cobblers arrived.[15] The other suspects were fishermen from Preston Pans who had abandoned their boats in Sunderland and Newcastle and had returned to Scotland overland, passing through Haddington.[16] Although it is possible that neither group was the source of infection, it is certain that Haddington's strategic position on the Edinburgh road ensured that some traveller was responsible for its epidemic.

In England, outside the North-East, isolated cases of cholera represented the norm during the winter months. Conditions were unsuitable for cholera's spread, but as spring advanced itinerant travellers began to move from their winter quarters. Raphael Samuel has vividly recreated the life-styles of those who lived on the open roads during the warmer parts of the year. Ranging from the habitual wanderers of no settled abode who flitted from place to place to those who made frequent short trips into the countryside but kept regular winter quarters in town, these wandering tribes fulfilled the seasonal needs of the British economy for manual labour, in the fields in the spring and harvest time, in the town when there were labour shortages.[17] Whether they were hucksters or showmen, Irish workers for the market gardens of Heworth or the half-gypsy canal boatmen, as the days grew warmer they left their lairs and headed into the countryside. An additional guest on their travels in 1832 was *V. cholerae.*

Without doubt the wandering tribes acted as major transmitters of cholera in 1832. Even at the height of the epidemic the disease spread slowly, almost at walking pace. It also followed the main highways, out from London, for example, towards Oxfordshire, Buckinghamshire and Hertfordshire. The isolated case which occurred in Dudley in March was that of a travelling German. His friends walked onto Worcester, where they were quarantined and closely guarded.[18] The first cases in Edinburgh were people who had been wandering in the already infected areas of Haddington, Tranent and Musselburgh. One was a ballad singer, another a rag and bone man.[19] In York the first case was of a boatman who, before falling ill, had spent several days ferrying vagrants from cholera-infected Selby across the Ouse for the York races.[20] Cholera reached North Staffordshire in June via a man of no settled abode who was found sick and drunk in Tunstall. He had previously been in Northwich, where cholera had broken out on 27 May.[21] In Worcester, the first case in July was of a rag collector living in the Pinch, a notably filthy part of the city.[22] Rag collecting was to become a notoriously dangerous trade, for it entailed extensive travelling together with the risk of handling infected clothing.

In the Midlands the bargemen of the intricate canal network did much to spread the disease in the summer. The first case in Warrington was of a bargemaster who had recently visited Winsford, where cholera existed but which the local medical profession had diagnosed as English cholera. The poor man was hastily buried, 'like a dog' according to one witness. A boatman from Shardlow brought cholera to Wolverhampton in mid-June. And the first three cases in Birmingham were of two boatmen and one of their wives.[23]

The annual fairs and wakes held during the summer were also major factors in the spread of the disease (August and September being the months for the traditional 'wakes' weeks in the Potteries and Lancashire).[24] Many of the wayfarers' itineraries were planned so that they could sell their small wares in as many of the fairs as possible. The authorities were aware of the danger from travellers and permission was given for the annual fairs in both Bristol and Wednesbury to be cancelled if the public health was felt to be threatened.[25] Even when fairs were held the threat of cholera cast a gloom over the proceedings. The June fair in Denbigh coincided with cholera's arrival. One observer, Daniel Jones, noted,

> How different the appearance of the people in this fair than in any other fair seen before in this generation. The country people make haste to return to their homes, fleeing as from an armed force of enemies. The fickle youth now chastened, their features changed, fearing the shafts of death with every flicker of an eyelid and everyone marvelling and wondering why we have been saved, and so many cut down.[26]

Cholera also cast a pall over the Reform Bill celebrations in many towns. At Holywell and Sheffield the first cases coincided with the celebrations.[27] In York, the pro-Reform magistrates suggested that the customary illuminations should be dispensed with and that the money saved should be given to the cholera hospital fund. In Plymouth, 10,000 people, representing the trades of the town, marched through the streets in celebration. The next day, cholera broke out.[28]

The spread of the disease reinforced the received conviction that the wandering tribes were a menace and danger to society. Under the Old Poor Law attempts had been made to regulate their movements, including the 1824 Vagrancy Act. But they failed because of an inadequate administrative machinery, ineffective police enforcement and because of the British economy's need for a mobile and versatile workforce. The letter of the law went frequently unobserved, but in 1832 rigorous attempts were made to solve the vagrancy problem. In that year 15,000 vagrants were committed to prison, compared with 7,000 in 1825.[29] It is possible that in the depression year of 1832 more vagrants were on the move; nevertheless, there is abundant evidence that in the year of cholera public opinion was more vigilant and suspicious of the wayfarer.

The normal procedure under the vagrancy laws was for the overseers of a parish where relief had been sought to send the applicant back to his place of settlement. Alternatively, they could relieve him for a day and then had the power to eject the applicant from the parish. With the threat of cholera being spread in 1832, neither method of dealing with wayfarers was suitable. In January 1832 the Central Board of Health had advised local authorities not to return vagrants to their place of settlement.[30] In Edinburgh the local board of health argued that it was of the 'utmost importance to the community . . . that the wandering of beggars and vagrants in a state of destitution, should as much as possible be repressed'. They should be fed and housed but kept in the parish until the disease abated.[31]

Such a procedure, however, not only increased the rates but also invited an outbreak of cholera in one's own parish. It was preferable to prevent vagrants reaching town in the first place. Schemes to further this aim were in the air from the time Sunderland became infected. In Blythe the local authorities debated whether to prevent vagrants staying in common lodging houses, while in York it was suggested that vagrants should be herded into an isolated house until the state of their health had been ascertained. Neither proposal was legal, nor was the decision of the Nairn board of health to hire 'retired military privates' to help in the suppression of vagrancy. During the fair in Beith late in August 1832, ten resident pensioners stood guard at the outskirts of town from dawn to dusk repelling 'unlicensed hawkers and confectioners'.[32]

It was the Edinburgh authorities who acted most decisively outside the law. They set up sanitary cordons on the roads to Haddington and Musselburgh to halt vagrants.[33] Not only was this illegal, it was also against the spirit of the government's recommendations (and, indeed, their own), because it did not actually prevent the poor from travelling. Fear of contagion spurred on the Edinburgh authorities. The local board was mildly contagionist,[34] but the mass of the inhabitants were strongly so.

> The Edinburgh folks are stark mad on contagion; they out-Herod Herod in their belief in its omnipotence, and fool, liar,

idiot, are profusely showered by its press on all who entertain a contrary opinion. They seem determined to be not only twice as religious, but twice as contagious as other people; they will have two fasts, and they have contagion of double strength.[35]

How strongly casual wayfarers were discouraged throughout the country in 1832 probably depended on the strength of local fears of contagion. Towns on tramping routes or on canal and river networks tended to act with the most initiative against wanderers. In Manchester, for example, two inspectors watched the canal boatmen coming from infected towns, but trampers were allowed in unmolested.[36] In April, all boats arriving in Doncaster from Goole were inspected, while in Burslem local inhabitants were urged to help the local constables arrest tramps. And in Cornwall the inhabitants of Mousehole erected a barrier across the road leading to the infected town of Newlyn. The barrier remained in place until a Newlyn woman threw some infected clothing over it in an attempt to spread cholera amongst Mousehole's population, with whom at that time there was bitter rivalry.[37]

Whatever the means resorted to, the local authorities must have at least implicitly sanctioned illegal measures. In many places, open support was given by the local ruling class. On 24 August 1832 an inquest was held in Exeter on John Vicary, an itinerant vendor of sweetmeats. The Captain of the Watch testified to stopping a cart at 3 a.m. one morning, suspecting that it carried infected bedding. The three men on board admitted having with them Vicary, who had fallen ill in Dawlish. Vicary died soon afterwards and the three men were arrested. At the inquest one of them, a Dawlish constable, claimed that three local parish officers had ordered him to carry the sick man back to Exeter. The gentlemen concerned were Robert Leeson, a Dawlish JP, William Hall, a Royal Navy captain, and Richard Ferris, brewer, coal dealer and overseer of the poor. The Exeter jury found them guilty of manslaughter. All three subsequently went into hiding, but at a later trial they were acquitted of the charges.[38]

Attempts to take the sick back to their place of settlement were supplemented by pressure being put on common lodging-house keepers. In Norton, East Yorkshire, for example, two women whose houses were frequented by 'strolling beggars and tramps' were sent to the workhouse and their houses shut up. Another man was refused permission to take in lodgers, and he was set to work by the parish.[39]

The wide range of evidence, covering communities of all sizes both sides of the border, demonstrates how widespread the threat from vagrants was felt to be in 1832. Action, whether to stop vagrants from arriving or to hasten them on after arrival, stemmed primarily from fear of their possible infectiousness, but also from an unwillingness to add to the poor rates. The Central Board, though faced with local initiative contrary to its recommendations, did not change its policy in 1832, and no action seems to have been taken against illegal local activity. On only a single occasion did the Central Board consider interfering, when a vast number of Irish congregated in Port Patrick to await transportation back to Ireland. The Board wanted to give them free passage on the Post Office packets (presumably to get rid of them), but the Treasury refused permission.[40] In every other case the local authorities were left to their own devices. As the number of vagrants imprisoned increased in 1832, it can be assumed that this was seen as an effective deterrent, although it increased the chances of cholera outbreaks in houses of correction. Neither government policy, which was sensible but ineffectual, nor local action could prevent wayfarers disseminating cholera in 1832.

According to the Official Cholera Returns of Great Britain, there were 71,508 cases of cholera and 26,101 deaths in Britain (excluding London) between October 1831 and December 1832. The total population in 1831, was 16,537,000, which suggests that, given the total number of people at risk, the epidemic was not very severe. But cholera was reported to have broken out in only 397 towns and villages in Britain, whose total population numbered 3,798,000.[41] Using this figure as the number *truly* at risk, the morbidity (sickness) rate from cholera outside London was 18.8 per 1,000 and the mortality rate 6.87 per 1,000. These figures certainly suggest that within certain areas cholera made a significant impact. In particular, the data suggest that cholera was more destructive in the small towns and villages of Britain than in the larger industrial cities. Table 2.3 shows the mean

Table 2.3: Cholera Morbidity and Mortality Rates, England and Wales, 1831–2

Population Size (000s)	No. of Districts	Morbidity per 1000	Mortality per 1000
<2.5	100	26.3	8.2
2.5–4.9	65	18.6	5.5
5.0–9.9	59	13.0	4.4
10–19.9	31	19.1	6.1
20–39.9	23	17.9	5.8
40–79.9	8	20.9	6.4
80+	4	14.1	5.1

Source: Cholera Returns of Great Britain, PC1/108

Table 2.4: Morbidity and Mortality rates, Scotland, 1832

Population Size (000s)	No. of Districts	Morbidity per 1000	Mortality per 1000
<2.5	36	21.0	8.7
2.5–4.9	37	15.8	6.4
5.0–9.9	23	19.8	8.2
10–19.9	4	33.8	14.8
20–39.9	4	16.2	8.4
40–79.9	2	15.3	9.3
80+	2	23.7	11.9

Source: Cholera Returns of Great Britain, PC1/108

morbidity and mortality rates for towns and villages in England and Wales. Table 2.4 gives the same information for Scotland. In both, towns and villages have been arranged according to population size, using the criteria of B. T. Robson and C. M. Law.[42] For England and Wales there seems no doubt that when cholera struck non-urban areas (i.e. villages with a population fewer than 2,500) it infected and killed a higher proportion of people than in the towns and cities. In Scotland the picture is somewhat different, with the highest rates occurring amongst the towns with populations ranging from 10,000 to 19,999 (Dumfries, Falkirk, Inverness and Kilmarnock). But the rates for Glasgow and Edinburgh also exceeded those for the non-urban areas. The mortality rates in Scotland, indeed, are consistently higher than in England and Wales and this is, of course, reflected in the mean case fatality rates (see Table 2.5). Even in the small towns and villages of Scotland, where the numbers are large enough to compare them meaningfully with England and Wales, the case fatality rate was on average 10 per cent higher.

Table 2.5; Comparative Fatality Rates, England-Wales and Scotland, 1832

Population Size of District	Fatality Rate % England-Wales	Scotland
<2.5	31.1	41.4
2.5–4.9	29.7	42.0
5.0–9.9	33.9	41.2
10–19.9	31.9	46.0
20–39.9	32.4	52.0
40–79.9	38.2	61.0
80+	48.6	52.0

Source: Cholera Returns of Great Britain, PC1/108

At first glance it is remarkable that the inhabitants of the smaller villages in England and Wales were more at risk than those in large towns. After all, cholera is famous primarily for its role in publicising the social defects of the large urban conglomerates in the nineteenth century. There are, however, several possible explanations for this apparent paradox. First, morbidity rates were more liable than mortality rates to under-registration, especially in the larger towns where it is likely that many cases occurred in areas beyond the influence of the local boards. The smaller towns and villages had fewer ghetto areas and this made the hiding of cases more difficult. Such an hypothesis, however, does not solve the problem on its own. Such evidence as is available suggests that the local boards in the large towns did act conscientiously if not always with efficiency. Neither does it explain the higher mortality rates in the villages, for it is unlikely that even in the biggest towns many cholera deaths could have gone unrecorded.

A more fruitful line to follow is that the morbidity and mortality rates are biased towards the smaller villages by the use of the total population figures for the larger towns. The urban rates are based on distorted population figures. The key to this lies in the dispersion of cholera in the larger towns. If cholera had been spread evenly, it would be valid to use the total population figure. But if cholera occurred in pockets, raging fiercely in some parts but leaving others untouched, then the total population figure would not convey accurately the number of people *truly* at risk.

The existing evidence suggests that in the larger towns and cities cholera was not widely dispersed in 1832. Robert Baker's famous *Cholera Plan of Leeds* shows that the main impact of cholera occurred in one (admittedly large) section of the city. Baker noted that amongst one-half of the population, who lived in paved streets with drainage facilities, there were only 245 cases. Amongst the other half, 1,203 cases occurred.[43] Similarly in Exeter, although there were cholera deaths in all but two parishes, 'the disease, as an epidemic, chiefly occupied the south-western quarters of the City'.[44] In York too, the main force of the epidemic was concentrated along the river banks and in the lower-class area of Walmgate. Cholera was also localised in Gloucester, Hull, Manchester and Wolverhampton.[45] It is surely significant that two exceptions to cholera's seeming fastidiousness were Liverpool and Bilston. From the arrival of the disease in the former in June it did not confine itself to one locality but could be found all the way from Kirkdale to Toxteth Park. Similarly, in Bilston at the epidemic's peak, cholera 'was literally sweeping everything before it, neither age, nor sex, nor station escaping'.[46] Both towns had the highest morbidity and mortality rates for their respective sizes in 1832, suggesting some connection between localised epidemics and relatively low death rates.

To explain the lower mortality rates in the large towns by reference solely to the proportion of their populations truly at risk is not enough, however. Reference must also be made to the critical role water supplies played in spreading cholera in 1832. In the larger towns water supplies came from a variety of sources. In York household water was drawn either from wells or directly from the rivers Ouse and Foss (which were used as a natural sewage disposal system). In Exeter there were numerous private wells, an ancient conduit, a few public pumps and the waterworks. But as these failed to produce a sufficient quantity of water, 'Much of the water used was . . . laboriously obtained by dipping it from the river or adjacent streams.' In Bradford, water carriers supplied the greater part of the population, while in Leeds, household water was obtained from a number of wells but also from the pestiferous river Aire.[47]

Thus, although the water supplies in the large towns were capable of gross contamination, they were also varied. In the smaller villages, however, most of the population depended either on one main pump or on the river, if the village was close to one. Once the water supply was grossly infected, nearly the whole population would be at risk. In the larger towns this was not necessarily the case, except perhaps for the riverside inhabitants who used the river as a water supply. If one regards the cholera epidemics in large towns as being a series of little epidemics close together with particular sources of water acting as focal points, then the relatively higher morbidity and mortality rates in the smaller towns and villages become explicable. In most of the large towns there were pockets where cholera ravaged extensively; in the smaller villages, there was only one 'pocket', the whole community.

The critical importance of water supplies leads on to another question: why in 1832 did some large towns, suffering from the side-effects of industrialisation, remain relatively free from cholera? The most surprising example of this phenomenon was Birmingham which, with a population of 147,000 had only thirty-one cases and twenty-one deaths in 1832. Other towns were equally fortunate. Derby had only thirty-two cases and sixteen deaths; Bolton, twenty-six cases and twelve deaths; Halifax, one fatal case; and Preston, nine cases with six deaths. No returns were received from Blackburn, Bury, Oldham, Rochdale, Huddersfield or Leicester.

While it is possible that the Central Board of Health was deliberately kept in ignorance of cholera outbreaks in these towns, it is more likely that they did escape cholera in 1832. A report that cholera was raging 'most dreadfully' in the Preston House of Correction appears to have been groundless,[48] and although it is possible that some cases went unreported in Bury and Huddersfield, it is doubtful that the local authorities deliberately concealed information from London.[49] Bury had only two fatal cases in 1832 and Huddersfield township no more than a few. It was in the small villages around these two towns where cholera spread and they were outside the jurisdiction of the local boards of health.[50] Moreover, the Central Board required information only if a widespread epidemic broke out; sporadic cases did not have to be reported.

It is fairly certain, therefore, that most of these towns were spared cholera in 1832. If an epidemic of widespread proportions had occurred, it would surely have received some attention at the time. There was, after all, little economic motive to hide cases by mid-summer. The government certainly had no regulations which might have convinced the local authorities that it was in their economic interests to keep cholera cases a secret. The movement of cloth was never forbidden; even the transportation of rags, on which the shoddy trades depended, was permitted.[51]

What, then, was the basis of these towns' immunity from cholera in 1832? How can Birmingham's good fortune be explained when in the summer of 1832 the smaller townships around it suffered terribly from cholera? Further north, both Oldham and Rochdale, linked to Manchester by the canal network, also remained free of the disease. It was not as if environmental conditions in these towns were significantly better than in some of the towns which suffered more severely from cholera. The *scale* of nuisances and overcrowding was obviously smaller, but this alone cannot explain their immunity, as much smaller non-urban villages were devastated by cholera in 1832. At Bamburgh in Northumberland, for example, twenty-three out of a population of 417 died, while in the agricultural village of Blackthorne, Oxfordshire, twenty-two died from a population of 400. Indeed, if we accept as unbiased the evidence on which Edwin Chadwick drew when writing his *Sanitary Report* in 1842, it could be argued that in many respects the cholera-free towns differed very little from those badly hit. The Manchester Statistical Society, for example, found that in 1,512 out of the 2,755 dwellings visited in Bury, more than two people were sleeping to a bed.[52] Of Halifax the local Poor Law Medical Officer wrote in 1842,

> Deplorable state of dwellings in certain quarters of the town. Irish lodging houses for vagrants and trampers of the lowest description and most abandoned habits. Want of attention in clearing away offensive matters in sewers, cesspools, privies, pigsties etc surrounding the houses... Compulsory draining and purifying of cottages much wanted.[53]

Such evidence, however, should be used with some caution. Chadwick, for very good reasons, was essentially a propagandist and only used evidence which suited his purposes. It is noticeable that he used little evidence from the towns under discussion, which suggests that they may indeed have been less filthy than one would have expected. If his use of Birmingham is taken as an example, it can be seen that although he does mention the town's comparative freedom from fever (because of its excellent drainage), he quotes only those parts of the local report which support the theory he is promoting. He quotes at length on the state of the common lodging-houses, but fails to mention that in the newly-built courts of Birmingham, of which there were many, environmental conditions appeared satisfactory.[54]

His most significant omission, however, concerns the state of the water supplies. According to the Birmingham physicians who compiled the report which Chadwick used, 'The supply of water is ample, and pumps are to be seen in almost every court. At Lady Well, Smithfield and Deritend, the water is of a very superior quality.'[55] Lower down towards the river Lea the water was of poor quality, but water from the canals was described as 'fresh and good'. Pure water was, of course, the crucial factor as far as cholera was concerned. While Birmingham was almost certainly not so filthy as the inflated industrial villages which surrounded it in the appositely named Black Country, it did have much of the squalor associated with the consequences of the population expansion in the nineteenth century. Yet it could escape the cholera epidemic in 1832 with only a handful of deaths and was to do so whenever cholera reappeared.

Similarly, the real explanation for the Lancashire and Yorkshire textile towns' immunity from cholera does not lie with environmental conditions but primarily with their water supplies: whether they were free of continued contamination and whether they existed in sufficient quantity to deter the poor from using alternative, but easily accessible, polluted sources of water. Most of the towns and villages around the Pennines escaped because their water supplies came from the rivers and streams which flowed down from the hills. Rochdale, for example, was served by four reservoirs which ensured fresh and abundant water.[56] Other towns, such as Halifax and Huddersfield, had a considerable proportion of their houses supplied by piped water from local water companies.[57] The Pennine towns had supplies which were not only purer and faster running than most others, but were also free from contamination as they had not previously passed through other populated areas.[58] On the other hand, towns such as Wigan and Warrington on the Lancashire plains were further from the original source of their water and thus at greater risk. Moreover, being closer to the seaboard, they were closer to the major cholera focal points. They were predestined to suffer more than Rochdale or Halifax, not because of environmental conditions, but because of their geographical location. Although the Pennine towns were not totally immune to cholera, they were better placed to escape the disease than their counterparts on the plains. It is ironic that the Pennine streams, the value of which had stimulated the original growth of these towns in the eighteenth century and had been a direct cause of the need for the rigours and discipline of factory life, acted as a positive deterrent to one of the most formidable scourges which ever threatened Britain.

Similar considerations explain the consistently higher mortality rates in Scotland in 1832. Relatively more Scots died of cholera because the problems of obtaining an adequate and pure supply of water was greater in the Scottish lowlands than in the similarly densely populated districts in England. The sanitary reports which Chadwick used showed the inadequacy of water supplies in many towns. Outside the Highlands, where factors similar to those in the Pennine region prevailed, every region's water supply was open to gross contamination. In Tranent, situated to the south of the Firth of Forth where the population consisted chiefly of colliers, fishermen, farm servants and labourers, Dr S. Scott Alison noted that

> I do not believe that there is a house . . . into which water is conducted by pipes. There existed great difficulty on many

> occasions in getting water at all.... Last summer the supply of water was stopped for several months.... I know that many of the poor were, in consequence, reduced to the practice of using impure and unwholesome water.... When cholera prevailed in that district, some of the patients suffered very much indeed from want of water, and that ... people went into the ploughed fields and gathered the rain water which collected in depressions in the ground, and actually in the prints made by horses' feet.[59]

The village had at one time been supplied with abundant water from a spring which fed ten wells, but frequently the water was diverted into a pit. Out of a population of 3,620, there were 282 cases of cholera in 1832, seventy-eight of whom died.

Household water was also in short supply on the west coast of Scotland. It was noted that in Ayr 'the water is strongly impregnated with lime . . . Strangers find it unpleasant, and I believe horses which have not been used to it are apt to suffer when it is given them to drink'.[60] Although Ayr was better placed in terms of nuisances and overcrowding than many other towns, in 1832 it suffered 436 cases of cholera, with 190 deaths out of a population of 7,600.

Further down the coast at Dumfries the complete water supply came from one source, the river Nith, into which the sewers poured their contents.[61] The local sanitary report of 1841 stated,

> It may ... be said that the cholera prevailed to a greater extent in Dumfries than in any other town in Scotland. Its ravages were greatest in the closes and other ill-aired places, though it would be difficult to specify any external distinction in many of the quarters where it prevailed. The disease attacked many individuals of the better class, and residing in what are considered the better parts of town.[62]

As in Liverpool and Bilston, therefore, the Dumfries epidemic was ferocious and undiscriminating because of the lack of choice in water supply.

The absence of a regular supply of pure and uncontaminated water in Scotland meant that a large proportion of the population was forced to seek any available source, however polluted. Of course, it could be argued that similar constraints prevailed south of the border and indeed in some places they did, but it is noticeable that when Chadwick came to consider the question of water supplies in 1842, he relied considerably on evidence from Scotland. For England he cited information from London, Manchester, Bath and Newcastle-under-Lyme, but the rest of his information came from much smaller, non-urban areas where water was in short supply, but where also the population at risk was quite small. The evidence he cited for Scotland covered most of the populated areas of that country and involved a significant proportion of the total population. Given his purpose of accentuating the worst conditions in Britain, the preponderance of evidence from Scotland is striking.[63]

Other factors, however, probably also played a subsidiary role. John Snow was later to point out that the Scots habitually drank unboiled water (usually with their whisky).[64] The English, more content with tea, were less at risk because they boiled their water. Geographical factors were also important. Most of the infected towns and villages in Scotland were concentrated either in the lowlands or close to the sea. Whether cholera spread by means of wayfarers or seafarers, it had a more susceptible population close at hand, more capable of receiving repeated infections than the more widely dispersed English towns and villages. Moreover, as a greater proportion of the Scottish population lived in small towns and villages, their higher mortality rates were spread throughout the spectrum, from the smallest non-urban community to the largest cities. Until a start was made to ensure that contaminated sewage was kept away from the available water supplies, Scotland was bound to be more at risk from cholera than the rest of Britain. It was to take another epidemic, of much greater proportions, to develop an awareness of this critical factor.

Cholera's sweep through the provinces in 1832 demonstrates that it was particular in its choice of venue and victim. It did not automatically seek out and destroy the poor and depraved, especially in Scotland where the water supplies were less varied. In Haddington in January 1832 a local magistrate noted that 'formerly cholera's ravages were confined almost exclusively to the lowest orders, to persons who either from extreme poverty, filth or intemperance were rendered liable to disease, but that now individuals in the middle ranks had been attacked and many of them fatally'.[65] Included amongst them was the father of Samuel Smiles.[66] It was not impossible for the propertied to be among the first victims in Scotland. The epidemic in Grangemouth was regarded with particular horror because 'its first victims were persons in a respectable line of life and where whisky drinking could not be fairly laid down as a predisposing cause . . .'.[67] It is unfortunately not possible to determine whether cholera killed a similar proportion of all classes at risk in 1832. Data exists for the first victims in Sunderland and Manchester and for most of the victims in York,[68] but as the propertied classes tended to be infected primarily when the disease returned for a second time or towards the end of an epidemic, no satisfactory conclusion can be reached from the evidence.[69] It is significant, however, that where the disease returned for a second time (as in Newcastle, Glasgow and Edinburgh) or where it apparently struck the propertied classes severely (as in Dumfries, Paisley and Bilston), the mortality rates were abnormally high. By implication, in those towns where the mortality rate was closer to the mean, the middle classes were probably spared, except when there was little choice of water supplies.

Cholera's occasional preference for the propertied is only one aspect of its unpredictable nature, for it also failed to strike in some admittedly filthy areas. Filth *by itself* could not promote cholera. To reach epidemic proportions cholera required an unbreakable link between filth and water supplies. Where major water supplies are capable of being repeatedly and grossly contaminated by cholera-polluted sewage, mortality is heavy and widespread. Where water supplies are multitudinous, the epidemic is localised. As an indicator of social inequalities or social dislocation, cholera could not compare with the fevers, which relied predominantly on filthy conditions and overcrowding for their diffusion. Admittedly, cholera could in certain circumstances highlight the same conditions (it was appreciated in 1848–9 that cholera frequently occurred in areas ravaged by fevers). However, cholera's appearance was the result of polluted water; filthy conditions alone made cholera of little more than marginal significance. Certain social conditions were, therefore, accentuated by cholera only at second-hand. Massive population increase, for example, put an undue strain on available water supplies. By 1848–9 alternative supplies had to be used, however offensive to the senses, thus helping to explain why the second epidemic, unusually, was frequently more severe than the first. Violent in its impact when water supplies became polluted, cholera used unsatisfactory environmental conditions only as a secondary means of spreading throughout a community. This not only mitigated cholera's impact in 1832; it also rendered comprehension of its etiology less likely.

3

Cholera and the Environment: The Case of London

THE suggestions offered in the previous chapter to explain the comparative immunity from cholera of some of the larger towns in Britain in 1832 relied on the specific etiology of *V. cholerae* and, in particular, on its ability to multiply rapidly in sewage-contaminated water supplies. However, to assert that cholera's virulence in Britain in the nineteenth century was merely the result of major defects in the system of sanitation somewhat begs the question, for *V. cholerae* interacts with the environment in ways other than the water supplies/sewage configuration. It could and did spread by person to person contact, a fact which John Snow was later to point out.[1] The optimum conditions for cholera's spread are determined by specific aspects of local physical, human and socio-cultural environments. *V. cholerae*'s 'ideal' environment would be hot and humid weather, a water supply capable of being repeatedly and grossly contaminated by sewage, and a relatively poor population crowded together in insanitary conditions, without the means of keeping their homes clean or of preparing and eating food in hygienic surroundings. With such a configuration cholera can be absolutely deadly, whether or not modern therapy is available. In contrast, cholera is highly unlikely to spread quickly during cold, crisp weather, when there is a filtered and reservoired water supply free from the discharges of sewers, and where the potential victims possess a standard of comfort sufficient for them to live in reasonably spacious surroundings and to adhere to basic concepts of food and personal hygiene. In short, conditions existing in modern western society are not conducive to cholera's spread.

Between the two extremes of the 'ideal' and the modern there are of course many intermediate positions, determined by the relationship between the environmental, biological and socio-cultural variables. While for the epidemiologist it is probably enough to know that a society tends towards the 'ideal' end of the spectrum for action to be taken, for the historian, interested in the effects of early urbanisation and industrialisation, a clearer awareness of these relationships is necessary. George Rosen has written that

> The occurrence of disease in a given population at a specified time exhibits a characteristic pattern defined by causation, morbidity and mortality as related to age, sex, social class, occupation, mode of life, and, more generally, to the culture and psychology of a society. The pattern of disease which characterises any group of people is not a matter of chance. It is an expression of their interaction with their environment in its various facets, and from this viewpoint certain diseases or groups of diseases may be considered as most characteristic or indicative.[2]

The most characteristic diseases in the nineteenth century, wrote Rosen in an earlier article, were typhoid (enteric fever) and cholera.[3] If he is right and diseases, be they acute or chronic, in some way *characterise* the society in which they exist, then they must 'help illumine the socio-economic features of the world in which they do—or do not—occur'.[4] Heart disease, for example, is a characteristic of western man's essentially sedentary existence, his tendency to eat and drink more than strictly necessary for health, and his stress-provoking lifestyle. If cholera is regarded from a similar perspective, what characteristics of nineteenth-century society are most likely to be illuminated and, more important, what weighting should be given to each variable? It is highly unlikely that answers of any authority can be given to the latter question, considering how difficult it is to make similar judgements when dealing with modern chronic diseases. Nevertheless, some attempts should be made to answer this question, more particularly because the first cholera epidemic in Britain occurred at a time for which there are no accurate morbidity and mortality data. Moreover, the 1830s is still a period of controversy for those historians who are divided over the effects of industrialisation on the living standards of the British people. Originally seen in rather narrowly economic terms, the debate has broadened into an evaluation of the standard of *life*, in which non-economic factors, such as the quality of life and the quality of food and drink, have played an increasingly prominent role.[5] Equally problematic, but with even less concrete data available, is the debate over whether the industrial revolution encouraged larger families (and thus created its own workforce), or whether the massive population explosion from the late eighteenth century was essentially independent of industrialisation. Both controversies, which are to some extent linked, remain contentious, partly because of ideological differences amongst historians, but primarily because of the absence or inadequacy of the raw data. In this context the cholera epidemic of 1832 could be of some value, but it would be an overwhelming task to trace the environmental linkages promoting cholera's spread in every infected area of Britain.

The obvious solution is a case-study of a particular town chosen for its intrinsic merits and for the more mundane reason that abundant evidence is still extant. With this in mind, London has been chosen. It has the advantages of having a massive population at risk, of being the object of several sanitary reports in the 1830s, of having most of its raw statistical data still extant, and of being comparable with other capital cities in Europe. Its major disadvantage is that its economic and social structure remained virtually unaffected by the early stages of the industrial revolution. Nevertheless, its rapid population growth brought environmental problems similar to, and probably greater than, those occurring in the burgeoning industrial towns further north. Also, its pre-industrial social structure and its domination by non-industrial forms of capital, facilitate the task of comparing it with other capital cities in Europe, especially Paris. The ultimate justification, however, can be seen in Table 3.1, for there was a striking difference in the mortality rates of Stockholm, Paris and London.[6]

Table 3.1. Mortality Rates from Cholera in Three Capital Cities (per 1000)

Paris 1832	Stockholm 1834	London 1832	London 1849	London 1854	London 1866
21.8	43.0	3.4	6.6	4.5	1.9

The staggering difference between London's mortality rates and those of Paris and Stockholm raises two immediate questions: how reliable are the mortality data for London?; and did London ever come really close to fulfilling the 'ideal' conditions in which cholera could spread most effectively? Regarding the 1832 data in London, there is no doubt that in a very small number of instances parochial mortality rates were seriously underestimated. But even if only half of the total mortality in London was recorded, the discrepancy between Britain's capital and those of France and Sweden would still remain enormous and require explanation. The second immediate question, relating to cholera's 'ideal' environment, requires extensive treatment. Given the importance of the water supplies/sewage configuration, it seems sensible to begin by examining the sanitary condition of London in 1832.

Metropolitan London had seven Boards of Commissioners of Sewers in 1832, each possessing separate and independent jurisdiction within their own limits (see Table 3.2). Two of these, the Regent Street Commission and the Blackwall Commission, were of minor importance, the former being responsible only for one street, the latter being concerned primarily with the drainage of marshland. Each Commission enjoyed different powers because although all were bound by the Old Law of Sewers (23 Henry VIII), which concerned only surface drainage, they had, with the exception of Tower Hamlets, extended their powers by local acts of parliament. These took some account of the massive population changes which had occurred since the Commissions' establishment. Nevertheless, once they all faced the similar problem of large-scale human waste disposal, their autonomy made the sewerage system in London totally anachronistic.[7]

Partly owing to apathy and partly to their interpretation of their powers, efforts made to augment and ameliorate the system of sewers varied from area to area. Both the Tower Hamlets and City Commissions believed they could build new sewers. In the former's jurisdiction a sewer along Ratcliff Highway had been built in the late 1820s, and in the City 'full one-third of the sewers . . . had been made by us in the last ten years . . . in streets where sewers had never existed before'.[8] In Holborn, however, only old drains could be replaced and in Westminster the Commission claimed it could do no more than maintain existing

Table 3.2. Jurisdiction of the London Commissions of Sewers, 1832

Westminster Commission	
St Pancras	Marylebone
Paddington	Kensington
Chelsea	Hanover Square
St James	St Margaret/St John
St Martin in the Fields	St Anne Soho
St Paul Covent Garden	St Mary-le-Strand
Holborn and Finsbury Commission	
Bloomsbury	Old Street
Holborn	Shoreditch
Clerkenwell	Rolls Liberty
Islington	
Tower Hamlets Commission	
Bethnal Green	Whitechapel
Hackney	Shadwell
Stepney	St George in the East
Spitalfields	Limehouse
Bromley	Wapping
City Commission	
City of London	
Surrey and Kent Commission	
Battersea	St George the Martyr
Lambeth	Bermondsey
Christchurch	Rotherhithe
St John Horsleydown	Newington
St Saviour	Camberwell
St Olave	Clapham
St Thomas	Deptford

sewers.[9] Apathy was rampant south of the Thames. Three local acts gave the Commission power to construct main sewers, borrow up to £100,000 and levy a shilling rate, yet in 1831 they still refused to cleanse open sewers unless owners of adjoining property paid the expenses. Although by 1834 they had an annual revenue of £12,000, they left 'the crowded slums of Southwark, the squalid cottages of Walworth Common, the mean streets of Lambeth and the vile purlieus of Vauxhall without any effective system of underground drainage whatsoever'.[10] Defective sewerage and drainage were to be recalled in 1847 by three surgeons who lived in the Borough during the first cholera epidemic. Robert Hooper remembered the absence, or defective nature, of cesspools in the large parish of St George, Southwark. Matthew Wagstaffe, who had practised in Lambeth, Southwark and Bermondsey in 1832, recalled following the path of cholera through the low-lying, crowded and ill-ventilated courts and alleys bordering the river. With many of the streets below the high-water mark, he frequently had to wade through diluted sewage effluent. Edward Doubleday reminisced on the open sewers in Christ Church parish, around which the cholera was particularly severe. He recounted visiting homes in 1832 and being 'almost knocked down by the offensive smells'.[11] Sarah Roberts, the first cholera victim in the Borough, lived in a house which had remained unwhitewashed and uncleaned for twenty years; it had an offensive sewer running along the back.[12] Undoubtedly, the worst conditions prevailed close to the river, where the offensive ditches of Lambeth, Rotherhithe and Bermondsey co-existed with sewers which were 'the receptacle of all kinds of refuse such as putrid fish, dead dogs, cats etc . . .'[13]

Similarly, to the north of the Thames, those parishes closest to the river suffered from the worst effects of defective sewerage and drainage. In the parishes of St Margaret and St John Westminster, parochial investigators in 1831 found that 'by far the greatest proportion of these parishes is either without any common sewers at all, or that where they exist, they are from dilapidation, or other causes, wholly inefficient'. Even respectable thoroughfares such as York Street and James Street had no common sewer, while cellars in Vauxhall Road were flooded to a depth of two feet. Nothing had been done to prevent flooding, although owners paid the sewer rate. The district visitors concluded that want of proper sewerage was one of the 'greatest and most lamentable obstacles to the ultimate improvement of the comfort of the poor . . .'.[14]

Even the out-ward of the wealthy St George Hanover Square had sewerage problems. Abutting the river and low-lying, it was inhabited principally by the poor. But the rest of the parish was also affected to some extent, with the wealthy being confronted with the results of insufficient drainage on their own doorsteps. The ornamental ponds in Kensington Gardens and Hyde Park contained the drainage from an estate recently built north of the Uxbridge Road, while the Serpentine took the sewage of Kilburn, Paddington and Bayswater.

> It is indeed a scandal upon the greatest metropolis in the world, that the only place near it in which the public can bathe is an open drain to a populous district, the filthy bed of which, when disturbed by even a single bather, causes the most unwholesome and disgusting effluvia imaginable.[15]

In fairness to the Westminster Commission, it is right to point out that the rich frequently did not bother to empty their cesspools but dug another when necessary. The Chief Clerk of the Commission noted in 1847 that 'many of the best portions of the West End are literally honeycombed with cesspools'.[16] By mid-century the best parts of London were 'floating' on what Henry Jephson called 'cesslakes'.[17]

Further east in St Anne's Limehouse the drainage was 'very inefficient indeed; the sewers are for the most part uncovered, and are very small in size, and mere open ditches, or perhaps some of them may hardly be called ditches; they are more like kennels . . . and yet effect an extensive drainage'. Only six hundred of the 2,500 houses in the parish were on a sewer; even Three Colt Street, the principal thoroughfare in the southern part of the parish, had underground drainage for only one-eighth of its length. Some houses had cesspools, but when full, as happened in Whitechapel also, these were emptied into the streets.[18] The greatest nuisance in the parish, however, was the Black Ditch, a noisome open sewer which meandered from Spitalfields through Whitechapel, Mile End, Stepney, Poplar and Limehouse before discharging into Limekiln Dock.

> It is the greatest abomination which ever existed, in the midst of habitations and public ways, and is of itself sufficient to infect the whole vicinity. Such another filthy sewer in an open state does not exist . . . in any part of the globe. It is truly so black, that its course may be traced for many yards after it has mixed with the water of the Thames, which itself is not the purest of rivers.

The Black Ditch had recently deteriorated after the Tower Hamlets Commission had connected it to a new sewer stretching from Stratford to Ratcliff; below the connection the Ditch had become sluggish and full of rotting effluvia.[19]

The City Commission of Sewers, which had authority 'directly or indirectly, over nearly every one of the physical conditions which were likely to affect the health or comfort of the [City's] inhabitants',[20] faced problems similar to those of Tower Hamlets. Cesspools were emptied into the streets and there was a particularly difficult sewer, the River Fleet. More than £1,000 per annum had been spent on arching over the Fleet in the years before cholera arrived, the work being done piecemeal as each successive stage of the new Farrington Street was completed.[21] It was not, however, the stench which caused complaints, but the fact that the sewage in the Fleet flowed from the Holborn and Finsbury area also. During normal weather this helped to scour the sewer, but when a storm coincided with a high-tide on the Thames, the water from the Flood was pushed back flooding many of the surrounding yards and cellars. Improvements at the Holborn end and an increasing number of houses attached to the sewer had worsened these effects. At certain times, therefore, it was probably healthier to live without sewers than live close to one prone to flooding.

The one Commission which did not have a boundary with the Thames was the Holborn and Finsbury. They claimed to have built nearly six miles of sewers in the 1820s.[22] Nevertheless, the older sewers still presented difficulties, especially the ancient Cock and Pye ditch. This served St Giles and St Martin in the Fields and was meant to drain the Seven Dials area, but no one knew in 1832 whether it was still functioning. The improvements to the Fleet mentioned above were said to have speeded up the flow of the sewage and to have reduced unhealthy exhalations, but its reopening in 1832 was thought to be the reason for an outbreak of cholera in Clerkenwell prison.[23]

However, much of this region was totally without sewers. In St Giles, Francis Nugee, a slum landlord, had hundreds of people on his estate living without the benefits of sewerage; most of his tenants were Irish, 'not the most cleanly in the world'. In the High Street people were paying 3s 6d a week to have water pumped out of their cellars.[24] Most of the cholera cases in St

Giles were to occur in the infamous ghetto region behind the High Street known as the Holy Lands. 'Not one of the streets had a sewer, and no house a drain,' said a local surgeon.[25]

The same story can be told for the Liberty of the Rolls, a small ten acre precinct either side of the lower half of Chancery Lane. For this tiny area a remarkable document remains from this period, the minutes of the local board of health. Here, in graphic detail, can be seen in microcosm all the worst features of London life in the 1830s. The visiting committees of the local board of health were extremely thorough in 1832. Every house was visited, with very few exceptions ('Number 6, Lees Buildings where there was no admission and no. 7 the same with great impertinence'). Every complaint was noted.

> Complaint of the police never being seen in the Rolls Building also of persons watering against the corner of No. 10 on their coming out of the King's Arms . . . Mr Mainwaring . . . complains of the nuisance occasioned by the dung heap—at times there will be pails of blood thrown thereon and maggots by tens of thousands make their way into his cellars.

There were no sewers in the precinct; the inhabitants retained their nightsoil in their cellars for sale at a later date. Some of the larger streets had cesspools but there were frequent complaints that they stank. The first case of cholera in the Rolls was to occur in White's Alley in a house 'without furniture but a heap of filth is collected in cellar'.[26]

Even on the periphery of London pockets of nuisances existed. Indeed, wherever people congregated, nuisances developed. For example, in St Mary Stratford-le-Bow most of the three thousand population lived in two pockets along the side of Bow Road and along the Old Ford Road. The sewerage system was a series of meandering open ditches which were frequently blocked up. The result, as usual, was dung heaps scattered throughout the parish ('Ginger's dungheap ought to be removed'). Similar conditions prevailed in Tottenham.[27]

The main defects of the sewerage system in London in 1831 can be summed up as follows. First, extensive areas did not have the benefits of being on a sewer. Second, where sewers did exist, they were frequently defective. Even the minority of householders with water closets did not, therefore, necessarily rid themselves of their waste product. Third, cesspools were the primary means of sewage disposal in London, but frequently they were emptied only irregularly and sometimes straight into the street. Fourth, many of the sewers were open to the elements and were thus prone to obstruction. Thromboses in the arteries of the London sewerage system were commonplace, although it is fair to say that in the northern parishes steps were being taken to reduce this risk.

The filth which lay around parts of London because of these deficiencies was never satisfactorily cleaned away in 1831–2. The loudest complaints heard in London in 1832 were caused by the failure of the dustmen to do their job satisfactorily. The evidence for this is endless. Part of the problem was the practice of 'treating', common in both rich and poor parishes. In St George Hanover Square there was 'a very general complaint that the dustmen refuse and neglect to cleanse the dust holes and bins'. In the Rolls Liberty they complained of 'the dustmen not calling and actually refusing to take the dust away unless fee'd or treated'.[28] The dustmen were, however, only the last links in a very weak chain which stretched from the privy to (hopefully) the Thames. As effluent followed this chain towards the river, it liberally and gratuitously spread its favours through all sections of the population.

London, according to the surviving evidence, was a filthy city in 1831, bisected by open channels of refuse, cluttered with heaps of rotting ordure, while beneath the streets subterranean streams struggled to cope with the waste products of a million and a half people. Certainly, bad drainage and sewerage were endemic in most of the London parishes, particularly in the older parts which came under the old Bills of Mortality. The parishes bordering the Thames were the main sufferers, primarily because of their marginally lower level, which ensured that they had to contend with the drainage of the higher parishes, the effects of flooding from the Thames, and the mixing of effluent from cesspools with river water through substratum percolation.

However, in seeking an explanation for London's comparatively low mortality rate from cholera in 1832, one must discover the capability which sewage had for repeatedly and heavily contaminating the major water supplies. The provision of piped water to the metropolis was in the hands of eight water companies in 1832: the West Middlesex; the Grand Junction; the Chelsea; the New River; the East London; the South London; the Lambeth; and the Southwark. With the exception of the New River Company, which took its water from various springs and the River Lea in Hertfordshire, all depended on the river Thames for their water supply (see Table 3.3).[29] That did not mean, however, that each company's water supply was equally at risk from sewage contamination. Three factors influenced the degree of risk facing the water companies in 1832: filtration; the continuity of water supply; and the siting of the pumping stations. It is now known that water which has passed through a simple filter bed is not a good vector of *V. cholerae*. In 1832, however, only the Chelsea company used a filtering system and this was still in the experimental stage.[30] Settling reservoirs, although not so efficient, can also have an adverse effect on the micro-organism's ability to reproduce. If water is allowed to settle for several days before being pumped into the piped network, *V. cholerae* will be greatly weakened.[31] In 1832 four companies had reservoirs: the South London; the Chelsea; the Grand Junction; and the Middlesex. The other companies pumped their water straight into their networks.

The continuity of water supplies could also have played a part in determining cholera's spread. Robert Koch, the first man to isolate *V. cholerae,* argued that in certain circumstances an intermittent supply of piped water could have diminished cholera's power. He felt that

> One could easily imagine that they [*V. cholerae*], like other bacteria, occasionally adhere to solid objects, e.g. to the inside of a piped system, which will be the case particularly if the movement of the water is slowed down temporarily or permanently. They can then perish at the place where they have settled down. . . . Generally speaking, the unequal movement of the water in a piped system must exert a considerable influence on the transport of the cholera bacteria and for this reason alone one pipeline may bring many and another few of the organisms to the corresponding houses.[32]

This view is of considerable importance because in 1832 water was supplied by the water companies only intermittently. The New River Company, for example, supplied water to the City

Table 3.3. Suppliers of Piped Water to the London Parishes 1832

Company		
New River Company	St Giles	Holborn
	St Martin	Islington
	Rolls	Clerkenwell
	City	Old Street
	Strand	Covent Garden
East London Company	Spitalfields	St George in East
	Bethnal Green	Poplar
	Shoreditch	Stepney
	Whitechapel	Limehouse
	Wapping	St Mary Stratford
	Shadwell	St Botolph Without
Chelsea and Grand Junction	Hanover Square	Chelsea
	Kensington	Fulham
	Paddington	
Chelsea Company	St James	St Margaret/St John
	St Anne Soho	
West Middlesex Company	Marylebone	
West Middlesex, New River, Hampstead	St Pancras	
Southwark Company	St George Martyr	St Thomas
	St Olave	St John Horsleydown
	St Saviour	
Lambeth Company	Christchurch	Lambeth
South London Company	Newington	Bermondsey
	Camberwell	Rotherhithe

of London between the hours of 6 a.m. and 6 p.m. on alternate days. It is just possible, therefore, that all the queuing and scrambling for water from stand-pipes which was a feature of working class life may have been worthwhile, if the water which eventually arrived was as a result less contaminated. However, one drawback of an intermittent supply was that continued unequal pressure of water in the pipes tended to crack the joints or, in the case of wooden pipes which were in some cases still in use, split them open.[33] This would have increased the possibility of a water supply becoming contaminated by seeping sewage after it had left a reservoir.

The third factor influencing the degree of pollution in the piped water supply was the siting of the various pumping stations along the Thames. Of importance here is their proximity to the major sewer outfalls: the closer they were, the greater the chance of gross contamination. All the major outfalls of the metropolis entered the Thames between the Black Ditch in Limehouse and the King's Pond sewer near Vauxhall Bridge. Only three pumping stations drew water from between these points: those belonging to companies supplying the parishes south of the Thames. Indeed, the Southwark Waterworks Company drew its water from a point immediately opposite the Walbrook sewer outfall at London Bridge. There can be no doubt that water companies supplying South London ought to have been most at risk from cholera in 1832.

This does not mean, however, that the other companies' water was free of pollution, although this was claimed by three of the companies before a parliamentary select committee in 1828. Independent experiments had indeed shown that the West Middlesex's water was the least polluted by 'organic material', it being the 'purest of all . . .; bright, clear, without taste or smell, but having a few fibres floating in it'. The Chelsea Company's engineer disputed this conclusion, claiming that his filtration process had greatly improved his water supply. 'The Thames has a taste, according to the season, of animal or vegetable matter, and filtration seems to deprive it of the whole of that, and we cannot discover it after it has passed the filter bed.' In a similar vein, the Grand Junction Company argued that although sewage did pass their pumping station, it did so only intermittently. Pure water could be assured if the pump was used at specified times of the day. The company chairman boasted that 'Not one drop of water that has ever been as low down the Thames as Vauxhall Bridge, ever returns; it is true, that the river Thames receives the drainage of London, and it is also true that the river Thames flows by Hammersmith; but it is not the same Thames.'[34]

The validity of these claims is doubtful for, although all three companies drew water from points above the main sewer outfalls, they were still subject to the tidal influence of the Thames. Similarly, the East London Water Company's pumping station on the river Lea was below the high-water mark of the Thames. Moreover, by 1832 conditions had deteriorated on the river. The pulling down of the old London Bridge in 1829, and the removal of its pillars which had acted as dams, had increased the tide's velocity and deepened the river's channel.[35] While the river bed was thus scoured more effectively, the solid contents of the river, and presumably also *V. cholerae*, were spread more widely. By 1834 it was accepted that the West Middlesex water supply had been 'triflingly affected' by the London drainage since 1829. Thus all the piped water supplies from the Thames were subject to some degree of pollution in 1832, pollution which most contemporaries agreed was gross. As Jephson was to write more than seventy years later, 'A river is always a great temptation to persons to get rid of things they want to get rid of, particularly when the things are nasty and otherwise not easily disposed of.'[36] Unfortunately, it was a temptation to which the Commissions of Sewers succumbed.

The proportion of people at risk from polluted *piped* water supplies cannot be satisfactorily estimated, because the companies supplied water to standpipes as well as to individual houses. But it is known that other sources of water were used and these too were subject to pollution. Wells are an obvious example. They were common on the north side of the Thames and were subject to contamination from the plethora of cesspools. In Clerkenwell, for example, 'The shallow well water of the parish received the drainage water of Highgate cemetery, of numerous burial grounds, and of the innumerable cesspools in the district.'[37] South of the river a general shortage of household water forced the inhabitants to use shallow wells which were subject to the tidal influence of the Thames. One alternative in Southwark and Bermondsey was to draw water from the extensive range of tidal ditches 'which were to all intents and purposes only open sewers'.[38] The most notorious of these were the ditches around Jacob's Island in Bermondsey, which both Dickens and Mayhew were later to publicise. Mayhew's description became famous.[39]

> As we passed along the reeking banks of the sewer [i.e., the tidal ditch] the sun shone upon a narrow slip of water. In the bright light it appeared the colour of strong green tea, and positively looked as solid as black marble in the shadow—indeed it was more like watery mud than muddy water; and yet we were assured this was the only water which the wretched inhabitants had to drink. As we gazed in horror at it, we saw drains and sewers emptying their filthy contents into it; we saw a whole tier of doorless privies in the open road, common to men and women, built over it; we heard bucket after bucket of filth splash into it. . . . We asked if they really did drink the water? The answer was, 'They were obliged to drink the ditch, without they could beg a pailful or thieve a pailful of water.'

These ditches were probably the most contaminated water supply in London. They were sluggish and, therefore, concentrated their effluent in a small area. Those who drank the water were probably more at risk than their neighbours who used the only other possible source, the Thames itself. Buckets of riverine water were the obvious source of supply for the poor who lived close to the Thames and could not use piped water.

Contemporary qualitative evidence and our knowledge of cholera's etiology suggest that in 1832 London's sanitary condition was variable. One must, of course, be wary of extrapolating from examples of particularly notorious plague spots to condemn whole regions, especially as much of the qualitative evidence comes from records which were lacking in precise objectivity. Witnesses before the various parliamentary committees frequently had a particular axe to grind. It is noticeable, for example, that the views on disease causation of every person examined before the Metropolitan Sanitary Commission in 1847 coincided not only with those of Bowie, the first witness, but also with those of Edwin Chadwick, the committee's major influence. It is known that such unanimity did not reflect the opinions of all the medical profession who practised in London in 1832. Evidence from the local boards of health's enquiries possibly suffer from a similar distortion. The district committees were engaged in a massive social survey, the objective of which was to uncover those aspects of London's sanitary condition which could give aid and succour to the threatening disease. It is worth noting that many of the London reports ended with the statement that the health of the poor was surprisingly good and that their habits were not so boorish as expected. It is as if the middle classes had not expected to find conditions which deviated from their preconceived notions and that these unexpected discoveries were added to the reports as an afterthought and not as part of their brief. Conversely, little or no evidence remains from some of the parishes, such as St Giles, St Clement Danes and Spitalfields, which were notorious for their overcrowded and insanitary conditions.

Caution, therefore, is necessary when using the qualitative evidence. Nevertheless, some conclusions appear to be valid. Without doubt the southern parishes bordering the Thames would have taken pride of place in any gazetteer of disgusting places. The combination of an inefficient and slothful Commission of Sewers together with unfiltered, heavily-contaminated water supplies was tailor-made for the diffusion of *V. cholerae*. Trailing slightly behind would come the East London parishes, drawing water from within the tidal influence of the Thames and suffering from widespread defective drainage. The riverside parishes were especially vulnerable.

> The whole of the coast, extending from St Katherine's Docks the entire length of High Street Wapping was very bad ... I know ... that the water for all domestic purposes was pumped into many of the houses from parts of the river where ... impurities abounded.[40]

Then would follow those northern parishes supplied, via filtering systems and reservoirs, from higher up the river. Probably least at risk from *V. cholerae* were those parishes supplied by the New River Company. Although the water arrived from Hertfordshire along a thirty-seven mile open ditch, which enabled it to be contaminated by surface drainage, cesspools, barges and bathers, it remained free of the noxious influence of the Thames. Pollution on a massive scale was, therefore, remote.

Table 3.4. Mean Morbidity and Mortality Rates, London Waterfields, 1832

Company	Mean density (per acre)	Morbidity (per 10,000)	Mortality (per 10,000)
Southwark	144.9	269.4	107.1
South London	17.7	106.6	46.4
East London	65.6	79.2	40.9
Lambeth	27.3	64.0	36.6
Chelsea	94.9	44.9	26.3
Chelsea/G.J.	14.7	53.5	25.9
New River	76.9	53.1	25.7

Sources: PRO PC1/108; Mins. Metro. San. Comm, 84.

The accuracy of the qualitative evidence is borne out by the data from the cholera epidemic in London. Table 3.4, showing the mean morbidity and mortality rates from cholera for the London water supply regions, highlights the massive differences between the rates for the Southwark Company region and those of every other. Beyond reasonable doubt, polluted water played a determining role in the spread of the disease in the Borough. That *piped* water was the main culprit is suggested by the much lower mortality rate in Christchurch Southwark which, except for its water supply, had the same socio-economic conditions as the Borough (see Table 3.5).[41]

The corollary of this is that piped water did not play such a crucial part in cholera's diffusion in the rest of the metropolis. Admittedly, Table 3.4 suggests cholera mortality outside the Borough to be in proportion to the degree of possible contamination of the piped water supplies which the qualitative evidence has shown. But neither the South London Company nor the East London Company regions could compare with the massive rates in Southwark. It would appear that either the pollution of alternative water supplies, or the transmission of cholera primarily by person to person contact, were more important for the rest of London. It is important to reiterate that John Snow believed some cholera outbreaks owed their transmission to the person to person syndrome. Indeed, he was prepared to argue that mortality rates below 53 per 10,000 in 1849 signified not the contamination of major water supplies, but the influence of poverty and overcrowding.[42] If Snow's analysis was correct, then mortality in 1832 should be regarded from a new perspective.

Undeniably, London was growing at an enormous rate during this period. Between 1821 and 1831 population increased by 246,000, a growth rate of 20 per cent. More than half this increment came from natural increase but the proportion of immigrants continued to rise.[43] Such a rapid increase must have put an added strain on the capital's social fabric; it certainly raised the demand for water by 25 per cent between 1828 and 1834. But the potential burden was lessened by the fact that physically London was growing outwards and not upwards. The highest rates of population growth in the decade before 1831 occurred in the peripheral parishes, with Kensington, St Pancras, Mile End, Lambeth and Camberwell leading the way. [44] In 1831 these still had relatively small mean population densities per acre, compared with the inner and older parishes (see Table 3.5).

It is true that these calculations do not take into account parks, docks and other open spaces, which distort population densities to some extent. Nevertheless, general social realities also help to explain the wide variation in parish densities. The high incidence of common lodging-houses in some regions is one factor to be stressed. They were to be found in St Giles, the out-ward of St George Hanover Square, St Mary-le-Strand and Covent Garden.[45] In St George Southwark in 1832 there were fifteen houses in Three Tuns Court, White Street, in which huddled 150 Irish. With the landlord in prison for debt, the poor had taken advantage of rent-free accommodation. In the Rolls, the most notorious dosshouse was the Red House, Chancery Lane, in which seventy people were sleeping in August 1832 when an arsonist set it on fire.[46]

Prominent amongst those seeking shelter in common lodging-houses were the Irish. Having migrated to London in increasing numbers in the 1820s, they numbered about 75,000 by 1841.[47] Their situation was unenviable: disoriented, demoralised and frequently unable to prove settlement, many were totally reliant on charity. They tended to congregate in particular parishes, partly for economic reasons, as in Lisson Grove Marylebone where building site work had been available, and partly for financial considerations, as in St Giles and Southwark, where the

Table 3.5. London Cholera Statistics, February to December 1832

Parish	Mean Density per acre	Morbidity Rate per 10,000	Mortality Rate per 10,000	Fatality Rate %
Paddington	12	58	20	34
Kensington	8	18	13	76
Hanover Sq	53	21	13	59
Chelsea	42	58	25	44
Fulham	5	14	5	33
St Marg./St John	57	66	38	58
St James	225	27	16	58
St Anne	284	24	16	67
Marylebone	82	42	18	43
St Pancras	40	18	11	60
Islington	12	16	10	65
Clerkenwell	149	30	14	46
Old Street	194	55	25	46
Strand	154	114	32	29
Holborn	230	45	12	28
St Giles	212	119	53	45
City	206	50	29	58
Rolls	268	97	41	42
Covent Gdn	200	58	35	60
St Martin	92	25	14	54
Shoreditch	111	16	8	53
St Botolph	108	796	289	36
Whitechapel	192	137	92	67
Bethnal G.	82	50	25	51
Spitalfields	2256	110	51	58
Stepney	60	97	45	46
St George	167	58	32	55
Shadwell	136	113	58	51
Wapping	94	79	67	86
Limehouse	56	120	53	44
Poplar	15	103	57	55
Stratford	5	62	18	29
Hackney	9	2	2	100
Bromley	8	16	0	0
St Geo. Sth	140	180	74	41
St John	141	558	171	31
St Olave	181	230	119	52
St Saviour	142	327	131	40

Table 3.5 *continued*

St Thomas	182	295	206	70
Christchurch	178	62	25	41
Lambeth	24	64	38	60
Battersea	2	17	11	67
Newington	71	107	45	18
Camberwell	6	77	37	49
Clapham	9	27	17	63
Bermondsey	48	173	71	40
Rotherhithe	19	16	14	90
Deptford	9	47	28	66

Source: Mins. Metro. San. Comm. 84.

poor law authorities were lax and charities more common. In 1832, however, the Irish were only a fraction of the vagrants who swept into London, justifying the fears of many of the middle classes that the streets of the metropolis were full of beggars, any of whom could be carrying cholera.[48]

There was also widespread unemployment and distress in London, which added to the habitual casual, under-employed labour force huge numbers of silk weavers from Bethnal Green, Shoreditch and Spitalfields. In February 1832, 6,000 people were crammed into the Bethnal Green workhouse.[49] The weavers were in the process of rapidly descending the socio-economic scale; between 1824 and 1848 their standard of living was to drop dramatically as a result of foreign and home competition, the over-extension of the labour market and the demands of under-cutting manufacturers. Cholera was to occur when distress was at its height; when 'disease, want and misery [had] increased to a most alarming degree', and when typhus was spreading through the slums.[50] In St Giles, experienced philanthropists discovered misery on an unprecedented scale. The St Giles' District Visiting Society, whose territory included the Holy Lands, informed the Home Office that at least a thousand unfortunates required immediate assistance. This was confirmed by one of the Central Board of Health's inspectors. Greville was shocked. 'A population more calculated to spread the present pestilence can scarcely be conceived,' he wrote.[51]

When cholera struck St Giles in 1832 it killed 280 people (mortality rate 53 per 10,000), most of the victims coming from the Holy Lands. Considering the acute distress which prevailed, mortality was slight. Nevertheless, it was far greater than in the other parishes supplied by the New River Company and significantly higher than the region's mean. In St Giles it was not piped water causing the damage, but local and particular social realities. In only one other part of the New River waterfield did comparable mortality occur—the Aldgate part of the City of London. But here too it was probably not the piped water at fault, but the pernicious influence of the famous, and in 1832 contaminated, Aldgate pump. Confirmation of this comes from the precinct of St Botolph Without Aldgate, which did not receive water from the New River Company yet suffered a massive cholera outbreak at the very same time as that part of Aldgate within the City became infected.[52]

Only the West Middlesex Company region had a mortality rate lower than the New River's in 1832. This company supplied Marylebone alone, a spacious parish where a combination of pure water and a relatively low mean population density per acre diminished cholera's virulence. Disturbances in the parish in 1832 suggest that the disease was most destructive in the Irish neighbourhoods.[53] Westminster and West London suffered only marginally more than the New River region. While it is likely that some deaths went unrecorded,[54] the low mean mortality rates are confirmation of the purer water supplied by the Chelsea and Grand Junction companies. It is significant that the highest mortality occurred in the combined parishes of St Margaret and St John. Their proximity to the Thames probably encouraged many to take their water direct from the river or from wells subject to substratum percolation. The piped water in the parishes was, moreover, open to contamination after passing the filtering system. The 1831 Westminster survey reported that 'For the first ten minutes after the supply was turned on, nothing but stale and offensive suds escaped from the issue—owing, no doubt, to the neglected state of the surface drainage, combined with some defects in the pipes.'[55]

The South London and the East London Company waterfields had higher mortalities from cholera in 1832 than anywhere outside the Borough. For the former, a possible failure to record deaths in Rotherhithe[56] and the use of a settling reservoir diminished total mortality, which may otherwise have rivalled Southwark's. The variation in mortality in the parishes supplied by the East London Company, with the highest rates closest to the Thames, suggests that the direct drawing of water from the river, or the pollution of local wells by river water, may have been the primary means whereby cholera spread. The exception, Whitechapel, may be explained in the same way as St Botolph. A well, or wells, possibly with the same source as the Aldgate pump, could have become grossly contaminated and thereby raised the mortality rate to ninety-two per 10,000.

A tentative conclusion, therefore, is that in very large parts of London in 1832 cholera's progress was dependent either on the pollution of *local* sources of water or on person-to-person contact. Piped water probably played a variable role but by and large it was not subject to the *gross* and *repeated* pollution by sewage necessary for cholera to spread both widely and virulently. Moreover, the dispersion of London's population over an ever larger area diminished the force of the person-to-person syndrome, while the considerable number of wells north of the Thames, and beyond its influence, increased personal choice. Where water was in short supply, as in Southwark and Whitechapel, the inhabitants were given the Hobson's choice of water which was undrinkable or no water at all. Mortality was consequently increased. Only in Southwark, with its undiluted sewage masquerading as drinking water, and its densely-packed and poverty-ridden population, did *V. cholerae* find its 'ideal' conditions for spreading in 1832.

The doubling of the metropolitan death rate in 1849 must be seen with the scenario of 1832 in mind. Between the two epidemics London's mean population density per acre increased from 34.5 to 50. Most of this increment occurred in those parishes (now Unions) outside the old Bills of Mortality. Moreover, important changes in the siting of some pumping stations had occurred. The Southwark and Vauxhall Company, formed by a merger between the Southwark and South London companies, had moved their station to Battersea Fields, half a mile above Vauxhall Bridge. The East London Company had moved further up the river Lea, beyond the influence of the tide. Both the Grand Junction and the Lambeth, the former having moved to

Brentford, had established large settling reservoirs. These changes may well have mitigated cholera's virulence in 1849, if the Thames had not, in the meantime, become even more pestilential. A larger population, of course, meant more sewage to contaminate the Thames, but it was not this alone which doubled the death rate. Much of the blame must fall primarily, and ironically, on Edwin Chadwick's sanitary policy of 'No filth in the sewers—all in the river.'[57] For Chadwick, the policy of flushing all London's filth through the sewer network was only a second-best solution to the sanitary problems facing the metropolis. Ideally, he would have preferred channelling the sewage onto agricultural land, to be used as manure. Failing this, he encouraged the Sewers Commissions to flush their filth into the Thames.

> Admitting the expediency of avoiding the pollution [to the Thames], it is nevertheless proved to be an evil of almost inappreciable magnitude in comparison with the ill health occasioned by the retention of several hundred thousand accumulations of pollution in the most densely-peopled districts.[58]

At the peak of the epidemic in August 1849, 5,743 cubic yards of sewage was entering the Thames each week, enough to explain why London suffered so severely that year.[59] In the peak months for cholera in 1832 (July and August), 2,602 deaths were reported; in August and September 1849 there were 10,895.

Table 3.6 sets out mortality rates for both 1832 and 1849 in some of the London parishes. The first significant point to note is confirmation that in 1832 the Southwark region suffered most severely because of *piped* water; their mortality rates in 1849 were not very different from 1832 (see Section A). However, those parishes such as Christchurch, Newington, Bermondsey and Rotherhithe which were not in the Southwark waterfield in 1832, but which were being supplied by the Southwark and Vauxhall Company in 1849, had a greatly increased mortality. Even allowing for some under-reporting of cases and deaths in these parishes in 1832, the changes are striking. A change in the siting of the pumping station had made little difference, because untreated sewage was still being pumped straight into the network.

The evidence from the New River waterfield is more difficult to interpret (see Table 3.6, Section B). All the parishes, with the exception of St Giles, suffered more severely in 1849. All had become marginally more overcrowded since 1832. Obviously, the water supplies in this region had become more polluted, but the significant point is that the mortality rates, compared with those south of the river, still remained relatively low. Although capable

Table 3.6. Comparative Mortality Data for Selected London Parishes

Parish	Mortality Rates (per 10,000) 1832	1849
Section A		
St Saviour	131	147
St Olave	119	180
St John	171	174
St George	74	172
Christchurch	25	166
Newington	45	144
Bermondsey	71	169
Rotherhithe	14	207
Section B		
St Giles	53	53
St Martin	14	37
City	29	64
Strand	12	36
Holborn	12	35
Islington	10	21
Clerkenwell	14	19
Old Street	25	34
Section C		
Bethnal Green	25	91
St George	32	42
Whitechapel	92	65
Stepney	45	47
Poplar	41	71

Sources: PRO PC1/108; Report on the Epidemic Cholera, 1850.

of pollution, the New River water was still purer than the water taken from the Thames. St Giles' static mortality rates may possibly be the consequence of the slum clearances of the 1840s.

The pattern in the East London waterfield is confused. Mortality was uniformly high, but while Bethnal Green's mortality rate nearly quadrupled, Whitechapel's diminished by a third. Grinding poverty does not seem to have been the crucial factor here; more likely, as in the massive 1866 outbreak, the East London Company may have been taking water from two sources, one of which was more polluted than the other.[60] Nevertheless, water from the Lea does not seem to have been so disastrous to the health as water from the Thames in 1849.

A general factor explaining increased mortality in the metropolis in 1849 is the larger proportion of the population receiving water from the companies into their homes in 1849. Competition amongst the water companies for trade in the 1840s, and the propaganda aimed at developing a 'sanitary frame of mind', had raised doubts as to the purity of well water which might have been polluted by cesspools or graveyard drainage.[61] The chances of a population escaping cholera, therefore, diminished as the 'sanitary idea' advanced. Because of an unfortunate order of priorities, established by a belief in the simplistic filth theory of disease, long-term sanitary progress was achieved only at the expense of short-term devastation. While it is true that, as far as typhus was concerned, the sanitarians achieved their goals in spite of a faulty ideology, their influence on cholera was negligible. Indeed, they helped to establish those 'ideal' conditions whereby cholera could be most virulent.

However, London's mortality rate of sixty-six per 10,000 in 1849 still pales into insignificance when compared with the mortality rates of Paris in 1832 and Stockholm in 1834. If one accepts that polluted water supplies constitute the greatest risk to health, then Stockholm's abnormally high mortality must be explained in this way. Stockholm's topography is the key to any explanation. Situated on a number of small islands, the city was served by numerous sources of water, but all were at risk from sewage pollution. A high proportion of the population had easy access to this water; once *V. cholerae* established itself, a devastating epidemic was assured.

Paris' higher mortality rate must be explained in different

terms. First, the French capital was more overcrowded than London (94 per acre compared with 34.5). Unlike London, it had not expanded outwards when population rose, but upwards and inwards. Overcrowding on this scale could only have aided cholera's spread by person-to-person contact. Moreover, a concentrated population meant concentrated sewage, and the Parisian sewerage system was defective. According to Louis Chevalier,

> The spread and layout of the sewers were no longer adequate for the population's requirements. Both the main encircling sewer—which took the rainwater and household slops of all the districts between it and the banks of the Seine at one end and the drainage of the northern faubourgs at the other —and the sewers on the southern slopes—which were entirely separate from the main sewer and flowed into the river through twenty-one outlets, the chief being the Amelot sewer, the sewer at Popincourt slaughterhouse and those at Petit Musé, the Grève and the rue de la Tannerie—were overtaxed, especially the Amelot.[62]

Although it cannot be said conclusively that the Parisian sewerage system was more defective than London's, it certainly had a more baneful effect on the water supply. Work had progressed on obtaining a supply of water from the Ourq canal by 1832, but the supply was still intermittent. It has been estimated that each Parisian received barely seven litres of water a day, while each Londoner received sixty-one. There were only 217 street taps in Paris in 1832 and very few houses had piped water supplies. Moreover, and this is the crucial point, the Parisian poor were prejudiced against the Ourcq water, although this was the only filtered supply in the city. With so few street taps, the average Parisian either had to buy his water from the commercial taps (there were thirteen in 1840), or he took water directly from the Seine which, with its twenty-one sewer outfalls, received sewage over a wider area *and was not tidal.* But even if the Parisian water supplies had not been so polluted, the higher mean density per acre would have ensured higher mortality in Paris than in London. 'Paris', wrote Chevalier, 'seems suddenly to become darker and unhealthier, crushed by its mass, stifled by its own respiration, transpiration and excreta.'[63] The evidence from the cholera epidemic suggests that this could not have been said of London in 1832.

Paris needs to be researched more fully before this comparative analysis can be confirmed, but it does help to put the London cholera epidemics into perspective. Massive population increases on their own are not necessarily conducive to cholera's diffusion if they can be spread over a wider area. In 1832 London still had room to expand; by 1849 it was rapidly filling up. By the time it was bulging at the seams later in the century, cholera had been controlled by the relatively simple expedient of providing a pure water supply. But the process whereby this occurred temporarily gave *V. cholerae* an advantage. It was not so much a change in London's socio-economic conditions which aided and abetted cholera, but administrative contrivance based on false premises. Nuisances by themselves could not seriously affect cholera's incidence; much depended on what the nuisances consisted of. Rotting organic matter may be offensive and a breeding ground for some harmful bacteria, but ironically these bacteria were more powerful than *V. cholerae* and killed it. Only when the nuisance consisted of the dejecta of cholera victims or carriers could it become a danger to the public health. It is salutary to remember that London was in less danger from cholera in 1832 than it was to be during its first period of regeneration under the sanitarians.

4

The Medical Police at Work in 1832

In one respect cholera's arrival in Britain in October 1831 heralded a change in government thinking about public health. The essential quality of the new Central Board of Health was its professionalism, reflected above all by its medical team of Major R. Macdonald and Drs Russell and Barry, all of whom had seen and studied cholera in field conditions.[1] Their practical usefulness demonstrated that the influence of antiquated medical science had been shrugged off; professional expertise replaced status as the main criterion in public health. Another small part of the Old Society had been chipped away. Tradition and precedent had laid down the ground rules for when an epidemic disease threatened, but they had few solutions to offer once a disease was present in Britain. Fresh ideas and flexibility were needed to face what was a unique situation. But these ideas were still expected to be formulated within the parameters of custom, tradition and political continuity. As well as having similar duties to perform as Halford's board (except that they had to prevent the spread rather than the arrival of cholera), the Central Board was still expected to rely on the 1825 Quarantine Act for its legal authority. It was the imperfect nature of this Act which eventually forced the government into passing an Act for preserving the public's health.

The underlying continuity in principle was reflected by the first Order in Council issued by the new board, which laid emphasis on the importance of local boards of health. Traditionalist and localist orthodoxies concerning the role of the State were stressed in a three-tier system consisting of the Central Board, district boards (covering the whole town) and subordinate divisional boards (covering individual parishes within a town). All sections of the local ruling elite were to be represented on the district board, while the divisional boards were to consist of a resident clergyman, a number of substantial householders and at least one member of the medical profession. The Central Board was to send new information and recommendations to the district boards, which in turn acted as clearing-houses for this information, at the same time sending back to the central authority the divisional boards' reports from the grass roots. The system was to be permissive and was to emanate from local, voluntary initiative. The Central Board was to act only as an advisory co-ordinating body; while decision-making was to remain in the hands of the local ruling class. Recommendations were to be deliberately left vague so that the local boards, with their wealth of local knowledge, would be able to extemporize more effectively.[2]

The Central Board's objective was to establish 'a general and combined system of sanative (sic) regulation, which in case of necessity may be acted upon throughout the country. . . .'[3] This was certainly innovatory, for although local boards of health had been established in the past during times of emergency,[4] there had never before been a policy of establishing a *national* and *uniform* system of public health bodies. Such a system was essential because of the widely varying and unsystematic administrative structures which already existed in the localities. Each community relied on governing bodies which had evolved out of its own individual history during previous centuries. The administrative area was the parish, in which the vestry managed poor relief, maintained highways and policed the village. As well as the 15,000 parishes in England and Wales, there were more than 200 chartered boroughs controlled by mayors, bailiffs and aldermen. But local government had failed to keep pace with the twin processes of industrialisation and urbanisation and in some towns without borough status there was a ludicrous discrepancy between the functions of the ruling bodies and the needs of a rapidly growing population. Manchester was a case in point. Power lay with the anachronistic Court Leet, the members of which were nominated by the steward of the Lord of the Manor. The chief officials were the Borough-Reeve and two Constables who were chosen annually from amongst the most respectable inhabitants.[5] Across the Pennines in Sheffield, there was in 1832 no municipal government, but local power was divided between five bodies, some ossified and some, like the Police Commissioners, of fairly recent origin. The latter had counterparts in many other towns where at various times the inhabitants had become frustrated with the antiquated system of local government and had paid for local Acts of Parliament which gave them some limited control of public affairs, usually in the fields of lighting, paving and policing. Local government was, therefore, a patchwork affair; 'no system at all, but a confused pattern of decay and growth'.[6] Placed in this context, the desire for a national system of local boards of health in 1831 is readily understandable.

Throughout the epidemic it was government policy to fuse central guidance with local initiative, but the blend of the mixture varied at different times. At first it was a touch of central control with a large dash of local initiative, but within a matter of days, when the second Order in Council of 21 November was issued, an attempt was made to enlarge the central authority's powers. The determinants were first, that some parishes and towns very close to the seat of the disease had not established boards of health, and second, that the Treasury had decided to give some discreet financial assistance to afflicted parishes, but only if a local committee, established under Privy Council authority, existed to take responsibility for the money.[7] Accordingly, a degree of compulsion was added to the Proclamation. Local authorities were ordered to establish local boards if and when the Privy Council so decreed (in practice this applied only to parishes where cholera was already present). At the same time, some limited power over nuisance removal was given to the local boards, although they still had to work with the usual authorities such as the magistracy and were not allowed to interfere in areas which came under the jurisdiction of established local bodies such as Commissions of Sewers.

Unfortunately, even these tentative steps were soon found to be illegal, being outside the terms of the 1825 Quarantine Act. It was this Act alone which the Privy Council could use to deal with every aspect of public health at this time, but it only came into force if a disease entered Britain by ship from abroad and this was never proved in 1831.[8] Complaints from local boards in infected areas persuaded the Central Board to inform the Privy Council in January 1832 that 'in many instances the public authorities of the places threatened or attacked—on a mature consideration of their powers—have not deemed the said Orders in Council legally binding'.[9] A growing awareness of this was to have disastrous effects on the morale of the local boards of health which, in a remarkable response to the October Proclamation, had sprung up throughout the country. Towns and villages most at risk from cholera in the North-East acted most speedily, but coastal towns and villages in East Anglia were also quick to appreciate the threat. Others as far from the North-East as Plymouth, Portsmouth and Swansea also acted swiftly, as did many of the larger towns at risk from their large populations and poor sanitation.[10] In London, at least thirty parishes had established boards of health within weeks of the November Orders in Council being published. Such a response was an undoubted coup for the Central Board; the appeal to local patriotism appeared justified. Even the City of London, long known for its suspicion of central government, was prepared to work in close liaison with the Central Board from the outset.[11]

However, not all the localities had acted with the same expedition. Some districts far from the seat of the disease failed to establish boards because of the supposed healthiness of the inhabitants. During the last months of 1831 the Central Board could do nothing to prevent recalcitrant vestries remaining inactive if they were not in an infected area, but as a result some towns were to be caught out by the unpredictable nature of the disease. When cholera made its sudden sprint to the area around Edinburgh in December, many authorities, including Haddington where the outbreak first occurred, were totally unprepared.[12] Similarly, cholera broke out in one of the London parishes which had not established a board of health. Greville noted in his diary on 14 February,

> On Saturday we had account of one or more cases [in Rotherhithe]. We sent instantly down to inspect the district and organise a Board of Health. A meeting was convened, and promises given that all things needful should be done, but as they met at a public house they all got drunk and did nothing.[13]

From the very beginning, therefore, there were significant gaps in the national system of local boards of health.

For those keen and enthusiastic boards which were established, the abortive Proclamations of 21 November caused endless confusion and unfortunately resulted in the most energetic over-stretching themselves. At the very least they could, without undue strain, examine their town's environmental condition. This required neither help from the permanent local authorities nor financing, being dependent only on the willingness of public-spirited men to give up some of their leisure time. But any attempt to improve social conditions depended on the relationship between the boards of health and the various existing local authorities: the vestry; the improvement commission; and the sewerage authorities. For what struck the members of the local boards most forcibly on their perambulations was that many of the nuisances and much of the defective system of public health already (in theory) came under the jurisdiction of established local bodies. In some instances a working relationship with the relevant body could be forged immediately, especially as the vestry or town council was normally the body which established the boards of health in the first instance, but there were some exceptions. In Tenby, inhabitants complained that the mayor's obstinacy had prevented the formation of a board of health. Although the Under Sheriff of Pembroke found the complaint groundless, a running battle was still being fought three months later.[14] In York, the mayor, Lord Dundas, was accused of selecting the central committee members of the local board on a partisan basis. He denied the charge, but nevertheless allayed opposition by co-opting the offended aldermen onto the board.[15]

In so acting Dundas followed the Central Board's recommendation that all shades of opinion should be represented on the local board of health. While this no doubt helped to temper local opposition and reduce possible inter-authority tensions, it also led to the establishment of some unwieldy boards of health. The tiny Liberty of the Rolls, for example, had twenty-two members on its board in November 1831, one for every ten of its inhabitants. Birmingham, by contrast, had only nine members and Edinburgh thirty-five.[16] Although difficult to substantiate, it would seem that the type of vestry influenced the size of the local boards. In an open vestry rival groupings could not be disregarded, but in select vestries opposition elements probably could be neglected with impunity.

Nevertheless, even if all the local authorities were represented on the board of health, ameliorative measures were not necessarily carried out. The key to action was not just communal zeal, but also an ability to raise finance and to overcome the obstacles presented by antiquated laws. For example, it was extremely difficult for a local board to abate a nuisance; Improvement Commissioners and Commissioners of Sewers could not be antagonised with impunity. The existence of a nuisance within a certain jurisdiction could not be dealt with; it could only be brought to the relevant body's attention. Whether action followed depended on the character of the local authority. In London, for instance, the Tower Hamlets and Finsbury Commissions of Sewers were amenable to approaches from local boards of health but across the river the Surrey and Kent Commission was positively obstructionist.[17] In other towns and villages in England, however, the local authorities could be helpful. In Exeter, the Improvement Commissioners supplied £1,000 to cleanse open drains and streets, build new sewers and provide water.[18] In Edinburgh, the scavengers, their numbers increased by thirty, carried off 3,000 extra cartloads of filth from houses and cellars by January 1832. The Police Commissioners, who paid the scavengers, also persuaded the magistracy 'not to weigh too nicely the amount of their powers' when they forced the local Irish to leave their pigs outside the city limits.[19]

But not all nuisances were subject to law. While rubbish in public places, such as markets and streets, could come under local Improvement Acts, those which existed on private property were subject only to the common law. It was in this sphere that many local boards of health found scope for action, for here they were not interfering in the jurisdiction of other bodies, but could act on their rights as private individuals. Unfortunately the process of common law was both irritating and inadequate. Any individual could apply to a local magistrate for a nuisance to be abated; an order would be made and served on the offender. Failure to abide by this order could lead to a fine, but the obtaining of such an order caused great personal inconvenience and it did not prevent the offender from allowing the nuisance to build up again. If this happened, yet another order had to be issued; this applied whether the nuisance was an overcrowded house, a heap of offensive ordure or straying pigs or chickens.

Nevertheless, local boards were better placed to deal with this process than an individual. They were well organized and probably had a better understanding with the local magistrates. This was certainly so with the Liberty of the Rolls board of health. A reminder of the 20 October Proclamation from the Hatton Garden magistrates caused the Rolls vestry to form a board of health in the first place. When the magistrates were asked what powers the board of health had over nuisances they replied that they would 'afford every assistance in their power and on reference to an Act of Parliament discovered there was scarcely a nuisance which could not be removed upon a summons to be applied for by the surveyors of the Liberty. . . '.[20]

In their exertions following this reassuring but too sanguine statement the Rolls board of health can be seen as a paradigm of all the other boards which tried to deal with private nuisances at this time.[21] In the first flush of zeal it was decided that all nuisance owners should be prosecuted immediately. This was rejected in favour of giving a warning to be followed by a summons if nothing was done. In some cases this had the desired effect. Mrs Lumley, the lessee of a string of brothels, did indeed clean her establishments (there was so much filth that huge mounds still remained after a week's work). But there were difficulties because most property in this part of the Liberty was let on leases for life, which meant that the owner (in the case of Lumley's houses it was the Bishop of Chichester), even if he was prepared to help, could not do so. The board had to warn each individual lease holder, who in many cases remained intransigent. Valuable time and the board's patience was lost. The task became too onerous and the board capitulated to the forces of inertia. After November 1831 no action was taken to prosecute recalcitrant nuisance owners. The board had to be content with a string of temporarily clean brothels off Chancery Lane.

Disillusionment came early to the Rolls board of health, but this was a pattern which sooner or later other boards were to follow.[22] At the root of their impotence lay the question of money. The failure to provide an adequate system of finance in this preparatory period was the Central Board's greatest failure. It had placed the whole onus for subsidising public health on individual and private charity. The district boards were to

> endeavour to remedy, by every means which individual and public charitable exertion can supply, such deficiency as may be found to exist in their respective districts in the following primary elements of public health, viz, the food of the poor, clothing, bedding, ventilation, space, cleanliness, outlets for domestic filth, habits of temperance, prevention of panic.[23]

The subscription was the traditional method of giving help to the poor and needy in times of emergency and has been called 'a principal weapon of the nation during the age of intermittent crisis'.[24] The only other source of local revenue was the poor rate, but the government could not order a rate to be levied for public health measures, nor was it clear whether the vestries could do so either. Even if they could, the poor in some areas would not benefit. This became known to the government from the moment cholera arrived in Sunderland. The township of Sunderland was divided into three socially delineated parishes in which the inhabitants paid a rate only for the upkeep of their own parish poor. In the poverty-stricken and overcrowded *parish* of Sunderland the rate was paid by a small proportion of the total population, who themselves were no more than small traders and 'incipient speculators'. Moreover, even labourers, when they felt economically secure, tended to leave Sunderland for the comparative comfort and high elevation of middle-class Bishopwearmouth. It was a struggle, therefore, to keep the poor from the brink of starvation even in the best of times. There was certainly no surplus for a subscription. The same problem arose when cholera reached the tiny villages and townships on the east coast of Scotland and the eastern parishes in London. In typhus-stricken Bethnal Green, for example, no voluntary funds could be raised from a population already crushed by the poor rate. The vestrymen could do no more than circulate 500 notices of advice to the poor and disinfect those workhouse wards where the inmates were suffering from typhus.[25]

This left government aid as the one possible source of finance for the poorest parishes (Barry's scheme for Sunderland, a uniting of Sunderland and Bishopwearmouth and the imposition of a joint rate, was obviously impractical during an emergency). As a Treasury Note of 14 November demonstrated, government was prepared to help distressed areas, but only grudgingly and as a last resort when local exertions had failed. Its unwillingness to intervene with financial aid showed its essentially traditionalist and moralistic outlook. Government officials feared that if central financial aid became widely known, 'the bonds of attachment', as Southey called them, which made the rich responsible for the poor and which prevented social dislocation, would snap.[26] Although government money was sent to Sunderland in 1831 when Barry returned horrific reports of the scenes he had witnessed, the government inspector on the spot, Lt Colonel Michael Creagh, kept the donations secret, 'lest it might have the effect of keeping individuals back and leading other towns to expect similar assistance instead of taking care of their own poor'.[27]

Charity, however, still had a possible role to play in those larger areas where there was a greater social mix. There the local boards of health used the money as if they were independent charity societies. Between November 1831 and February 1832, 16,000 articles of clothing were given to the poor in Edinburgh. In York a sub-committee led by George Hudson, the future railway king, spent £150 on blankets and shoes. In the city of London between £2,000 and £3,000 was spent on bedding.[28] The houses of the poor were also whitewashed. This was typical of charitable endeavour, the discovery of its usefulness having been called 'the most helpful fact in the philanthropic history of the eighteenth century'.[29] Charles Pearson, Chairman of the City of London board of health, bought one ton of chloride of lime (cheaply) on behalf of the board for distribution around the wards.[30] Whitewashing the houses of the poor gave a psychological boost as much to the givers as to the takers, acting as therapy for the beleagured local boards.

The establishment of food kitchens was felt to be another way of keeping cholera at bay. Eight were in operation in Edinburgh by February 1832, giving away soup and bread at a weekly cost of £250.[31] Like other charitable responses, this helped to allay the local boards' frustration caused by the failure to act constructively in other fields. It was a positive attempt to reduce the 'pre-disposing' causes of cholera, but at the same time it was not unique, only supplementing or supplanting those normal charitable activities current during the winter months.

However, once these measures were embarked upon, frequently it was found that traditional subscriptions began to dry up.

In Edinburgh, for example, where £1,500 was raised in November alone, subscriptions to the local board of health rose as the longer-established charities found theirs diminishing. It was not, therefore, a question of more money being spent on the poor in 1831; rather, the same amount was being allocated in a different way. As expected, the money was insufficient for the board's purposes, between £6,000 and £7,000 being needed just to keep the operation ticking over.[32] In York, attempts to re-channel money raised for the poor in Ireland into the board of health's coffers were thwarted by the Quaker Joseph Rowntree, who claimed such procedures to be illegal.[33] By the time cholera came to London in February 1832 hardly any local board had prepared temporary hospital accommodation for the sick. Not even the purses in St George Hanover Square were deep enough to pay for this outlay. Financial arrangements had thus broken down, even though most local boards had gone no further than organising traditional charitable activities. It was an alarming discovery. The customary method of maintaining social harmony and control had collapsed. It would take more than charity to solve the massive problems of the new urban environment.

As the realisation of their helplessness dawned on the local boards, a mood of pessimism and gloom enveloped the committees. This is reflected in the local boards' minutes for, after the upsurge of excitement and fear in November, interest began to wane. In Manchester the board of health was frequently inquorate by the end of November. By the turn of the year some of the London boards of health had ceased to function, while the local board in St Mary Stratford-le-Bow was meeting only once a month. Indeed, the system of local boards began to ossify almost as soon as it began. Partly this was owing to the illegal nature of the Proclamations of 21 November; the Central Board of Health informed the local boards that they should not act on the Orders. This left the boards with very little to do, once they had completed their rounds of the poorer quarters. Their charitable exertions could do not more than scratch the surface of the direct want and misery which was accentuated at this time by widespread unemployment. Temporary and congenital distress had coincided at the most dangerous time. A writer in *Blackwood's Magazine* in 1830 spoke of

Not merely that kind of want which must necessarily be found to some extent in all great cities, where disease and crime get huddled together in dark corners, and even common charity is scared away from those foul recesses in which all that is loathsome in degraded humanity rots and dies, in obscure despair. Not such want as this we speak of; but the decay of laborious decency, the misery of semi-starvation from want of employment of those hands which have never been employed in anything but honest industry, is even in the metropolis deplorably prevalent.[34]

To the credit of the Central Board of Health they had quickly become aware of the massive physical problems which beset the local boards, and from January they had insistently told the Privy Council that new legislation was indispensable. It is possible that they would never had been heeded if it had not been for the outbreak of cholera in London in February 1832. Some more cynical members of boards of health outside London noted that it took an outbreak of cholera in the city where Parliament was sitting for a Bill to be introduced. Robert Christison, Professor of Medical Jurisprudence and Police in Edinburgh University wrote in February 1832,

For months the pestilence raged at Sunderland, Newcastle, and their neighbourhoods in England, and in Haddington, Tranent, and Musselburgh, in Scotland, without recourse being had to any measures which deserve mention; but the instant that a few cases appear in the great centre of opulence, all is panic; assessments and additional powers are proposed in Parliament; national grants of money recommended; and every thing conceded to the terror of the metropolis, and the apprehension of popular displeasure . . .[35]

Christison had a point, for the Cholera Prevention Act was brief but had all the hallmarks of a panic measure. The core of the Act was

that it shall and may be lawful for the Lords and others of His Majesty's Most Honourable Privy Council, or any two or more of them . . ., by any Order or Orders to be by them from Time to Time made, to establish, and again from Time to Time, by any such Order or Orders, to revoke, renew, alter,

> and vary all such Rules and Regulations, or to substitute any such new Rules and Regulations as to them may appear necessary or expedient for the Prevention . . . of the spreading of the said Disease called the Cholera, or Spasmodic or Indian Cholera, in England and Wales or any part thereof, or for the relief of any persons suffering under or likely to be affected by the said Disease, and for the safe and speedy interment of any person or persons who may die of the said Disease.

The Privy Council had been given unlimited power in the field of public health, a fact appreciated by the government. Lord Althorp, introducing the Bill in the Commons, admitted that 'Undoubtedly . . . he was giving great and extraordinary powers to the Privy Council.'[36] The duration of the Act, until the end of 1832 or the end of the next session of Parliament, alone checked the Privy Council's power. No member of Parliament opposed this, the most far-reaching part of the Bill; an emergency obviously required emergency legislation. Even the philosophic radical Joseph Hume accepted its necessity, especially to 'enforce rigid habits of cleanliness'.[37] Panic was at the root of Parliament's haste to give absolute powers to the Privy Council. Knowledge of cholera's presence in the capital was enough for a Bill to be passed which potentially surpassed any other piece of centralising legislation in the century.

Ironically the Privy Council did not use its available powers immediately: regulations dealing with the environment, for example, were not made until 19 July. This was partly because of cholera's failure to spread throughout the country before the summer. Even in London the disease was relatively innocuous, apparently disappearing in May. This breathing space allowed the Privy Council time to gather its wits, but by July a new crisis had arisen. Not only did cholera return with great virulence to London but it also spread throughout the great manufacturing districts of the Midlands and the North. Its rapid diffusion pointed to a failure of local initiative to prepare for the epidemic. The result was the Proclamation of 19 July, a clear case of bolting the stable door after the horse had bolted. This Order differed from its predecessors only in the wider scope which it theoretically gave to the local boards of health. They now had the right to open and cleanse sewers and drains, remove nuisances from private property, establish burial grounds and pay for medical assistance for those sick at home. But, and this was the crucial point, the local boards could act only after the vestry had sanctioned their plans. Failure to get agreement meant going through the long process of writing to the Privy Council to obtain a Proclamation overruling the vestry. The machinery was too cumbersome for effective use during an emergency. Moreover, the local boards were not given any jurisdiction over nuisances which were the responsibility of Improvement Commissions or Commissions of Sewers. Nor could they enter and clean a house, or remove a nuisance unless the owner gave his assent. In purely sanitary affairs, therefore, the local boards were still effectively powerless.

Nevertheless, the local boards had some scope with the practical problems raised by cholera's presence in the community. Whether or not they were successful in this attenuated role is hard to estimate, because evidence remains for only a handful of local boards. The weight of material from the Privy Council and the Central Board of Health diminishes rapidly after the Central Board's daily minutes were discontinued in May 1832 (when, let it be noted, the disease seemed to have disappeared from London). Moreover, although some twelve hundred local boards of health were established in 1831–2, the minutes survive for only a fraction of them. Some of the minute books are incomplete, particularly those for the London parishes, which tend to become silent at the most important moment, when cholera is actually present. As all the boards whose minutes peter out were in London, it is possible that the special circumstances of the epidemic in the metropolis, with its two distinct phases, could have led to the breaking up of the local boards in May. They presumably reassembled at the end of June, for some minutes were kept in September and October, but for the height of the epidemic there is nothing. The possible reasons for this will be discussed later; suffice to say here that most of the extant source material is silent during the crucial phase. Any conclusions reached concerning the activities of the local boards in 1832 must therefore be tentative, especially when the rural parishes are discussed.

What, however, seems clear is that most of the boards faced similar problems and by and large they tackled them in a similar manner. Given their powerlessness over wider sanitary problems, most of their activities related to the practical objective of reducing the impact of cholera to a minimum. First and foremost, there was the need to isolate the sick from the healthy in temporary hospitals, but not, as Halford's board suggested, by compulsion. Also necessary was a reception house for those who were possibly in the incubation period, and a house of recovery for convalescents. Temporary hospitals were to be at the forefront of local board activity in 1832. At first, it was thought that the obtaining of a suitable house would be relatively easy, but this confidence was frequently misplaced. Manchester was a case in point. The local board sought two suitable establishments, one at either end of town. By mid-November they had drawn up a list of forty potentially suitable houses and factories. (This was one way in which the commercial slump was advantageous.) In December one factory was selected but, terms having been agreed, it suddenly became unavailable. Another factory was then leased, which eventually became the reception house, while two more were found to be used as hospitals.[38]

In Manchester hospital accommodation was found relatively easily because the leypayers had sanctioned the spending of the rates on them. But local feeling, raised by the prospect of patients arriving who were suffering from an infectious disease, was against the use of factories in populated areas as hospitals. Everyone accepted the need for hospitals, but no one wanted them on his own doorstep. In the larger towns, however, hospitals could not be established too far from the centre, for it was from here that the victims were most likely to come. Some inhabitants had, therefore, to suffer, but they did so not without a struggle, which involved the threat of writs.[39]

Similar feelings to those in Manchester were expressed in other large towns. In the City of London action was only taken when the disease was already in the metropolis. In haste the Lord Mayor offered a house in Abchurch Lane rent-free, an offer which was too good to refuse. But being close to the commercial area as well as to large concentrations of the poor, petitions of protest were sent to the mayor by bankers, merchants and the poor law authorities of St Mary Woolnoth (the last group probably fearing they would eventually have to foot the bill). Although the board of health agreed not to use the house, it became the major cholera hospital in the City during 1832 because the disease arrived before alternative arrangements could be made.[40]

The one generalisation which can be made regarding the provision of temporary hospitals in 1832 is that with financial backing and the tacit support of the local authorities, potential opposition could be withstood, at least in the larger towns. This was not necessarily so in the smaller towns and villages where subscriptions were fewer and the local bodies less pliant. In Ely for example, where 'a strong spirit of opposition, nurtured by a few individuals, has shown itself to the measures instituted by the Board for preventing the spread of cholera', the local board was still desperately seeking a suitable building three weeks after cholera had arrived. In Boston, where the vestry refused funds for the leasing of the most suitable building (a corn warehouse), the board of health had to make do with a storehouse.[41]

An enormous variety of buildings eventually housed the sick in 1832, ranging from bricked-off sections of workhouses to badly-ventilated and dilapidated houses close to bone-yards. Where they existed, local boards frequently tried to obtain barracks. William Pitt had ordered the erection of many during the French Wars and they were ideally located, being close enough to the main centres of population to overawe possible dissidents, but not too close for the troops to be susceptible to the contagion of radicalism. Unfortunately, the need to keep the troops free from disease was particularly pressing and thus permission to use them was always refused.[42] Some boards went further than they were legally entitled in their search for a suitable building. In Dumfries the board of health forcibly 'requisitioned' a house still under lease, while in Warrington it was considered whether to move 'certain families' from the town altogether and house them in sheds or tents made from tarpaulin.[43] In rural areas, hospitals were only infrequently established, probably because of the absence of a large concentrated population (as in the parish of Tardebigge); in such circumstances it was too dangerous and expensive to carry the sick to hospitals a considerable distance away. A hospital was established in Plympton after the disease had been raging for weeks, but here the disease had until then occurred in only one small hamlet.[44]

Contemporary evidence suggests that the provision of temporary hospitals was probably counterproductive in 1832. Nearly all the available data points to the cholera hospitals being truly 'the gateways to death' (see Table 4.1). Contemporary opinion supported these findings. It was not unpreparedness, callousness or ineptitude on the part of the hospital staffs which caused these strikingly different fatality rates, for patients on the whole appear to have been treated with compassion and humanity.

Table 4.1. Comparative Fatality Rates in Hospital and at Home, 1832

Town	Fatality Rate (%) Hospital	Home
Bristol	61.5	38
Liverpool	54	25
Wakefield	54	37
Sheffield	49	24
Leeds	47	37
Newcastle (Staffs)	37.5	18
Worcester	21	29

Source: Hospital rates, PRO PC1/111; Home deaths calculated from PRO PC1/108.

Admittedly it was probably preferable psychologically to be treated at home with one's family to nurse one, but medical attention there tended to be spasmodic. In Plympton, for example, although the local doctor and the incumbent were extremely conscientious, many of the sick could be seen only fleetingly as the doctor rushed off on another call.[45] Moreover, the insanitary conditions among which the poor lived were not conducive to survival. On balance, therefore, it was better to be cared for in the hospitals. The fatality rates were higher because in the main only terminal cases could be persuaded to enter hospital. The fears which hospitals aroused were caused by factors outside the control of the local boards. A major fear, that the sick would be murdered and their bodies used for dissection, was the result both of the Burke and Hare and Bishop and Williams murders which had occurred so recently and the movement for the passing of an Anatomy Bill. Some local boards tried to solve the root cause of these fears by promising that no postmortems would be carried out without relatives' consent and by allowing patients to be nursed by a member of their own family. Nevertheless, the sick poor continued to use the hospitals only as a last resort with the result that the doctors could do little by the time they were admitted. The hospital staffs were caught in a vicious circle: the sick poor would not be helped until the existence of the hospitals could be justified; but no justification could be found while the fatality rates remained so high. In the event, the hospitals, on which the local boards expended so much energy and finance, were unable to accomplish the aims for which they had been established.

The other major duty incumbent on the local boards during the epidemic stemmed partly from the failure of the hospital system. Where were the bodies of the cholera dead to be buried to prevent them becoming an additional risk to the living? The Central Board had recommended in December 1831 that the dead be buried as soon as possible, wrapped in cotton or linen cloth saturated with pitch or coal tar, and carried to the grave by as few men as possible. The funeral service should be held in the open air. The Central Board gave no further advice on this matter until 19 July, although privately they advised local boards to bury the dead within twenty-four hours. The 19 July Proclamation introduced a permissive system for burials, local boards being allowed to purchase a burial ground (using local rates) outside the town limits. Their doing so made it illegal for the cholera dead to be buried elsewhere without the local board's permission. Corpses now had to be interred within twenty-four hours of death.

As with the establishment of hospitals, the most severe problems beset the local board in the larger towns. An adequate burial ground, isolated from the mass of the population, was an expensive prospect. The cost of conveying bodies long distances was also prohibitive but, with the knowledge that the usual burial grounds were filled to bursting point, many local boards had seriously to consider buying a plot of land. Sheffield was one of the more fortunate towns. The Duke of Norfolk saved the ratepayers about £600 by allowing part of the local park to be used for cholera victims.[46] In York, money was saved by allocating part of the Corporation's lands (close to the present railway station). However, the local board was split down the middle when the

Corporation, arguing that their lands could not be alienated indefinitely, claimed that the burial ground could be used for other purposes after the passing of twenty years. This decision outraged many inhabitants (and the Tories), especially those who had had relatives buried there (the surviving gravestones show that some of the middle-class and lower middle-class dead were interred in this spot). The arguments subsided only after it was decreed from London that burial grounds had to be consecrated in perpetuity, a decision which effectively secured an eternal resting place for the dead.[47]

York had needed a new burial ground because of the unsatisfactory nature of those which already existed. In London the graveyards were in an even worse condition. Eleven years after the cholera epidemic Edwin Chadwick was to 'popularise' the disgusting conditions in the intramural burial grounds, but these conditions were already known to the authorities in 1832. Four of the district inspectors reported on the inner London burial grounds for the Central Board in January 1832. Apart from two small unconsecrated spaces, they could find no spare ground for possible cholera dead and concluded that more land was essential if mortality became exceptionally high.[48] In that there was a need for a general cemetery, to cater for all the London parishes, the issue belonged particularly to government. The Central Board consequently began to enquire after suitable sites. The exorbitant cost of land, which rose even further when it was learned that a cholera burial ground was being sought, left only one alternative, the purchase of seven acres at Kensal Green from the General Cemetery Company. The remarkable fact about this episode was that the Central Board wanted to buy the land, not to facilitate the burial of the poor cholera victims, but to give *the rich* an exclusive resting place. Almost as an afterthought the Central Board suggested that land on the outskirts of London should be sought for general interments.[49] There was to be a class dimension even in death. As it happened the purchase was never completed and the London parishes were left to their own devices, and by and large they did little or nothing. Land was, of course, at a premium, especially for the central parishes. Nevertheless, the City of London authorities did no more than consider the possibility of a new burial ground between October 1831 and February 1832; decided then to pay a reasonable sum for land outside the City but did not do so; and finally, as the second phase of the epidemic swept the City in July, began seriously to consider possible sites. Eventually land in Holloway was purchased for £4,000 but as the disease had declined in virulence by then it was never used. Holloway prison was later built on this site.[50] Meanwhile the cholera dead in the City of London were being buried in plague pits.

The major justification for separate burial grounds was the need to keep contagious corpses separate from the living; judged by this criterion the efforts of the local boards were a failure. It is a fair assumption that the majority of cholera corpses in 1832 were interred within the parish boundaries, and wealthy victims within the church vaults.[51] Even when separate burial grounds were found, often they were not outside the town limits. When in Manchester the local board tried to prosecute relatives of victims being buried in the churchyards, the magistrates refused to help because the new cholera burial ground (in the workhouse graveyard) was within the town's limits. An appeal to the Privy Council was rejected and thus potentially lethal bodies continued to be buried close to large populations.

The provision of hospitals and burial grounds were only two of the issues which the local boards of health tackled in 1832, but they were the most important and the most intractable. Given the contemporary justifications for them, neither were successfully dealt with. However, the local boards were not total failures; much of a temporary nature was accomplished. The establishment of reception houses for possible carriers of cholera probably helped to nip many small foci of infection in the bud. The use of expurgators to limewash infected houses had similar small-scale results.[52] The practical effects of nuisance removal were more limited, partly because in many places the drive to eradicate them came too early and partly because the local boards had neither the finance nor the practical means of working systematically (although where they had, as in Manchester, some slum areas were cleaned).[53] But overall the local boards failed. What was lacking was a strong and purposeful lead from central government. The absence of firm leadership kept the relationship between the Privy Council and the local boards tenuous throughout 1832. Only on very rare occasions, as when cholera arrived in London, did the Central Board of Health intervene decisively in local affairs. They did not even force every local authority to establish a board of health. Bathurst informed the Manchester board in May 1832 that 'Their Lordships have not interfered with the formation of Boards of Health in any towns or districts (sic) leaving them at all times to the spontaneous arrangements of the local authorities.'[54] Any relationship which existed between the localities and the central authorities was, therefore, on an *ad hoc* basis.

Indecision in Whitehall appears to have centred not in the Central Board of Health but in its parent, the Privy Council. The extant evidence, admittedly piecemeal, suggests that the Central Board was more willing to follow an innovative policy than the Privy Council, which still appeared to be steeped in the ideology and mentalities of the past. But throughout the epidemic the Privy Council, no doubt mindful of Halford's disastrous desire for autonomy, kept a very tight control on the Central Board of Health, which consequently never broke away from its purely advisory role. As a result the potential which existed in the local boards was vitiated by the absence of a coherent philosophy of public health at the centre. Rules and Regulations were issued, not according to a set plan, but because of sudden crises, which caused government policy to lurch forward intermittently.

The lack of long-term central planning was demonstrated by the role which the medical inspectorate was expected to play. These inspectors had potentially a very important function, for they could have been the means by which the central government penetrated the fortresses of localism. Gutchen has noted that,

> The key to the development of central supervision and control over local government lies not in the evolution of a system of centralisation, but in the struggle by the government to impose national, uniform, standards of sanitary administration within the framework of local autonomy.[55]

To achieve this an inspectorate, responsible to the government and not to the local authorities, was indispensable. But in 1832 the inspectors were given only a very limited role in the localities. They had two primary duties: to give advice and encouragement to the local boards; and to act as an alternative (and unbiased) line of information from the localities to Whitehall. They were not permitted to order the building of hospitals or the separation of the sick from the healthy. Nor were they sent into an area until cholera was suspected. Thus they were too late to have any influence during the preparatory period. Moreover, although the size of the inspectorate was quite large (sixteen at least) when compared with others which were to be established in the 1830s, they were too few to have more than a marginal influence when cholera spread rapidly through the country in the summer of 1832. It was not that experienced medical men were unavailable; rather, the Privy Council did not wish to antagonise local opinion by foisting central agents onto the local boards. It is true that in the early months of the epidemic medical superintendents had not been well received. They were, for example, unpopular in the small villages on the west coast of Scotland. One inspector found it impossible to find living quarters in Kilwinning and a man who offered him accommodation was intimidated into changing his mind. Local opinion here was moulded by the fear that the inspector would bring the disease with him,[56] but in Glasgow the local medical profession shunned the inspectors because they objected to any outside interference. One inspector, Thurston Caton, was unable to examine the records of the local cholera hospital, while Arthur, the principal government inspector in West Scotland, was 'not only insulted in words but threatened with an assault' by a magistrate in Helensburgh when he asked to inspect the body of a suspected cholera victim.[57] By April 1832 poor Arthur was at his wit's end.

> I have served more than thirty years in the army under difficulties and in times as eventful as has fallen the lot of the medical officer, but I have never experienced any service so unpleasant as the present. What between the hazard of the disease, the dangers of a lawless mob, the numerous perplexing references, the laborious extent of the responsibility and the unsatisfactory result of our exertions—I am extremely fatigued with the concern.[58]

Not only was the inspectorate expected to play no more than a minor role; it was also used as little more than a temporary expedient. The ephemeral nature of the whole exercise was confirmed by the inspectorate's dismissal as soon as cholera seemed to be waning. The four Scottish inspectors and eight of the twelve inspectors in the metropolis were given notice in April, although London was not officially declared free of cholera until 7 May. Admittedly, this was a period of acute political crisis and the government would have gained kudos by being able to publicise cholera's defeat, but nevertheless the unseemly haste in which the inspectorate was broken up demonstrated the temporary nature of its role and the Privy Council's inability to plan for the long-term. When cholera returned with increased severity in the summer, the Central Board, which had been unwilling to disband the inspectorate, had to fight for its re-introduction.[59]

With the inspectorate powerless and the Central Board of Health circumscribed by its dependence on the Privy Council, the local boards of health received little support when they came into conflict with the local entrenched authorities. Nor were they given much practical help if the dissension came from within their own membership.[60] Moreover, when local boards of health were in conflict over such questions as whether those who fell sick in a parish other than their own should be allowed entry into that parish's hospital, the Central Board refused to intervene. In London, each parish was regarded as an island. Only when the sick from the Houseless Poor Asylum were refused access to the local cholera hospital did the Central Board act, transferring them to the hospital ship *Dover* moored off Limehouse.[61] It is significant that action was not taken until a situation arose in which the Central Board could not be accused of interfering in the internal affairs of the parishes.

Central initiative was used effectively in only one sphere, that of finance. The Cholera Prevention Bill had been passed with the minimum of debate in February, but on the question of financing anti-cholera measures there had been a difference of opinion along party lines. Althorp had suggested at first that parish expenses should come from the poor rates initially and ultimately from the country purse, for he believed that as the whole country would benefit from the work of the individual parishes, it would be invidious to expect only the infected parishes to foot the bill. The underlying principle was still, however, that the localities were responsible for their own local costs. In contrast, Peel and Goulburn for the Tories argued that as county boundaries were arbitrary, and as the whole nation stood to benefit from anti-cholera measures, the charge should be accepted by the state and paid for out of the general fund. A national calamity required national remedies which superseded the rights and duties of the local authorities. Althorp and Poulett Thomson for the government rejected this suggestion (and with it the underlying principle) by claiming that it would lead to extravagance and the extinguishing of private charity. Eventually a compromise was reached whereby each parish would pay its expenses out of the rates and the government would reimburse the most poverty-stricken at a later date. The Privy Council was to decide which parishes were to benefit from the general fund.[62]

Powers were therefore given to the Privy Council to order local vestries to levy a rate specifically for the local boards of health, although a limit was set on local board expenditure (£50 on nuisance removal for example). Nevertheless, whenever a vestry refused to support the local board, the Privy Council issued an Order in Council against them. Usually, however, it came too late, for the local boards, fearful lest they might be left personally responsible for their debts, eschewed action. Moreover, the system did not help the poorer parishes, for it presupposed that the vestry could raise a rate in the first place. For some of the London parishes this was impossible. In Shoreditch, for instance, the poor rate was at its highest ever in 1832 and the vestry already owed £3,000 'on good faith as collateral'. In February 1832 the Shoreditch authorities asked the Central Board of Health for a grant, but the Treasury refused because 'it would break their rules and cause embarrassment and difficulties . . .'. The Central Board, more aware of the distress in parishes such as Bethnal Green and St Giles, wanted grants to be allocated, but the Treasury would only offer money on loan. Eventually, a grant of £2,000 was given to Bethnal Green (probably because the social conditions in that parish had recently been discussed in Parliament), but no money was paid over to the other distressed parishes.[63] Because of the absence of minutes after May 1832 it is not possible to discover whether other parishes tried to obtain government aid, but it seems unlikely. The London parishes were a special case because of their proximity to Parliament; other parishes did not present the same threat. Moreover, in their final report in December 1832 the Central Board of Health admitted that 'the great study of the Board has been to effect its measures with the greatest possible regard to economy'. While this statement does not preclude government aid in 1832, it is likely that financial frugality was achieved at the expense of many lives. The government had left its weakest and most helpless children to fend for themselves (sometimes against rapacious authorities), at the very time when they most needed succour.

They did so because they failed to come to terms with the possibilities raised by the introduction of a new authority (which they had inspired) in the localities. They sought and to some extent tapped a vein of enthusiasm in the localities but failed to find a viable role for it to play. Ever mindful of localist susceptibilities and failing to generate a sanitary ideology, they lost an opportunity of taking a vital step towards founding a permanent system of public health administration in Britain. It was not only a failure of nerve, but also a failure of vision. With the authorities transfixed by traditional modes of thinking, cholera was seen as a transitory phenomenon requiring only temporary remedies. Neither the disease itself, nor the social conditions which it publicised (and which many thought were the cause of cholera), had sufficient impact on the set attitudes of the central authorities to lead to permanent remedies. It is ironic that cholera, the most feared disease of the nineteenth century, was not so devastating as perhaps it should have been in 1832, for it did not jolt the government from its traditional and customary preconceptions.

5

Cholera, Medicine and the Medical Community

CHOLERA invaded Britain when the medical community was in deep crisis, both structurally and intellectually. In the eighteenth century, although there had been some progress in fields such as midwifery and morbid anatomy, medical science had failed to capitalise on earlier advances. At the end of the seventeenth century,

> All that seemed necessary ... was for medical science to continue steadily along the way of the physical disciplines, and for medical practice to follow closely after. A good start had been made in this direction by the end of the seventeenth century. Then a strange and tragic thing happened.... Medicine at first faltered, and then fell behind; physic failed to keep up with physics.[1]

Whereas the mechanical sciences had benefited greatly from Newton's synthesis, similar attempts in the field of medicine had resulted only in arid speculation and dogmatism. Far from reaching an acceptable synthesis, philosophical ventures in the field of medical science led to a myriad of conflicting theories, all of which needed to be taken with a large dose of 'logic' to become palatable. Long-running controversies erupted, in which the tone of debate became vituperative; dogmatic opinions undermined scientific discipline. Some demoralisation in the medical profession followed; it is not very surprising to find many medically qualified men at work in other fields of natural philosophy by the end of the eighteenth century.

Moreover, during the first decades of the nineteenth century, the twin processes of industrialisation and urbanisation had further undermined the antediluvian structure of the medical profession. The diffusion of wealth amongst a growing middle class had increased the pool of potential patients capable of paying doctors' fees; their living in or near the burgeoning industrial towns of the Midlands and North had placed them in areas outside the control of the two major medical institutions, the Royal College of Physicians and the Royal College of Surgeons in London. By 1830 a large proportion of the middle class was being serviced by doctors whose qualifications and experience varied greatly. The old tripartite division of medical men into physicians, surgeons and apothecaries, each with their own specialist functions, no longer conformed to reality. Instead, even in London there was emerging a new breed of doctor, the general practitioner, able and willing to prescribe medicines as well as act as surgeon, man-midwife and pharmacist.[2]

Such a development naturally caused tensions within the medical community. The old structure was based on a strict hierarchy of orders, into which it was impossible to fit the general practitioner, for he performed the functions of all three types of medical man. The cream of the medical community were the physicians, particularly the Fellows of the Royal College, who fought hard to retain their privileges and, above all, their high social status which, claimed one member of Halford's board of health, was a consequence of their sharing an exclusive education with the gentry at Oxford and Cambridge.[3] Holloway has argued, convincingly, that by supporting the Apothecaries' Act of 1815 the Fellows managed successfully to defuse the medical reform movements which had originated amongst the junior ranks of the profession early in the century. Although the Act increased the Society of Apothecaries' jurisdiction and augmented its powers, it also kept the hierarchy of orders intact and emphasised the low-status trade origins of the Society.[4]

In essence, the Act worked to block the social pretensions of provincial practitioners who eagerly sought a share of the growing middle-class market. Ian Inkster has recently used the concept of the 'marginal man' to help explain the difficulties facing those provincial medical men seeking social status. Writing of the medical community in Sheffield between 1790 and 1850, Inkster has stated that 'medical men were marginal twice over, for they were both provincials striving for individual status, and members of a profession yet in the making'.[5] He contends that practitioners attempted 'to legitimise their social and intellectual positions through social action', by membership of societies and by 'affiliation with identifiable (i.e. image-producing) religious and political movements'. Granted this to have been the case, it is clear that the onset of a new and dangerous disease offered an opportunity for practitioners to promote their social image by actually fulfilling a need, not in concerns such as mechanics' institutes which were peripheral to their occupation, but in medicine itself. It was a chance for practitioners to gain prestige both for themselves *and* for their profession.

The opportunity came at a most auspicious moment, for in 1831 the reputation of medicine was at a particularly low ebb. Apart from the long-term reasons mentioned above, three factors probably contributed most to the unpopularity of the medical profession. First was the knowledge amongst the educated lay public of some of the worst scandals which had ripped open medical society in the 1820s. Thomas Wakley, self-appointed defender of the general practitioner, played a central role in exposing the corruption, nepotism and graft occurring in the highest echelons of London medical society. Through the columns of *The Lancet* he had constantly harassed the Royal Colleges with a stream of invective and accusations, taking individual surgeons to task for operating in a slovenly and dangerous manner, and attacking the privileges of the elitist Fellows.[6] While his objective, to raise the status of the bulk of the medical community, was no doubt laudable, and while he had some public support (sufficient for juries to give derisory damages to his opponents in libel cases), in the short-term his exposures only brought medical men into disrepute.

Of more immediate consequence to the reputation of the medical community, and in the short-term extremely damaging, were the revelations concerning the Burke and Hare outrages in Edinburgh in 1828 and the subsequent discovery of gangs of burkers in London in 1831. An attempt to legislate against burking had failed in 1828 but in 1831, at the same time as cholera arrived in Britain and burkers were caught in London, a new Anatomy Bill was presented to parliament. The Bill would have reduced the threat of middle-class graveyards being despoiled, but it worsened the position of the poor, for it permitted local authorities to give up to surgeon-teachers bodies which remained unclaimed in public institutions such as workhouses and alms houses. Thus, although perhaps tempering middle-class attitudes to the medical community, the Anatomy Act (it became law in July 1832) reinforced popular feeling against medical men.[7]

The influence of the third factor underlying lay opinion on the medical profession is much more difficult to assess, for it involves the attitudes of patients to their treatment by medical men. It is by no means clear, for instance, what expectations the patient had when visiting a doctor, whether he expected a complete cure or was satisfied with some relief to his symptoms. Attitudes to hospitalisation suggest that the medical community was held in no great confidence, although hospital mortality was not so high as was once thought.[8] Hospital patients, however, were not drawn from the ranks of the middle classes, who were usually treated in their own homes. The social successes of the quack St John Long and of the phreno-mesmerist Dr John Elliotson suggest a lack of confidence in mainstream medicine at this time, possibly a consequence of the medical community's failure to fulfil the expectations raised by their claim to membership of a *scientific* community in the 1820s.

The doctor-patient relationship, the meeting of the lay world and medical science face to face, is of course a crucial factor for any understanding of the status of medicine. Was it capable of overriding the disastrous consequences of the scandals in the hospitals and the bodysnatcher scares? What it seems to have done is develop an ambivalent lay attitude to medicine, which distinguished between the personal and the institutional: the collective image of medicine was badly tarnished; the personal image of the individual medical man remained largely intact. Wakley was very aware of this ambivalence. In 1832 he wrote,

> The medical profession, *as a body*, commands but little of the respect and esteem of the people at large. As individuals, they are admired and beloved within the immediate range of their labours but . . . the profession, as a body . . . carries not with it the weight and force of national character which belongs to the profession of the law or that of divinity.[9]

Most medical practitioners concerned with the relationship between medicine and society must have had some knowledge of this ambivalence; this awareness conditioned their responses to cholera in 1832.

Medical response to cholera in 1832 was, therefore, influenced by three considerations: the desire to protect the community from an extremely dangerous disease; the need to maintain or increase lay support for medicine as a profession; and the wish, on the part of each medical man, to confirm or raise his position *within* the profession. The remainder of this chapter will be concerned with the consequences of these influences on medical activities in 1832, particularly with reference to theories of disease causation and therapy.

Before 1832 imported exotic diseases had not failed to become subjects of controversy in Britain although, owing to the absence of major epidemics since the last great plague outbreak in the seventeenth century, they existed as little more than potential sources of conflict. Broadly, a medical practitioner in 1831 could choose one or a combination of three traditional views of disease causation. The first was the theory of the 'epidemic constitution', a revival and extension of the Hippocratic theory which had gained considerable support in Britain through the agency of Thomas Sydenham in the late seventeenth century. The core of this theory was the conviction that the seasons of the year and the atmosphere were the main determinants of the nature of a disease. While these determinants caused a particular atmospheric condition suitable for the spread of a particular disease, they did not on their own explain variations in susceptibility amongst the population. Sydenham had explained this difficulty by reference to an hypothetical x-factor, peculiar to those infected: the development within them of an abnormal composition of humours. The specific characteristics of each disease would be determined by the particular interaction taking place between the personal x-factor and the two external factors.[10]

Sydenham mentioned 'contagion' only three times in his writings: when discussing plague, venereal disease and 'intercurrent and stationary' fevers. But early in the eighteenth century Richard Mead resurrected the doctrine of contagion, which had been developed furthest by Fracastoro in the sixteenth century. Concerned with plague, Fracastoro had argued that the disease could be transmitted in three ways: most frequently by the direct contact between the sick and the healthy; by coming into contact with infected clothing or goods; and, rarely, by inhaling an infected atmosphere. Mead, however, incorporated into this theory an x-factor, which he believed to be a chemical corruption of the atmosphere caused by *local* miasmatic exhalations. Local influences, although still secondary to the contagionist principle, became a significant part of his epidemiology.

These three factors, contagion, epidemic constitution and local miasms, were to dominate epidemiological thinking until the 1850s. But their importance fluctuated considerably between 1700 and 1850. By 1800 a general theory of disease causation was being promoted which laid increasing stress on the importance of local miasms. The doctrine struck firm roots in the United States, a consequence of the findings of Benjamin Rush and Daniel Webster in their study of yellow fever. Rush, a product of Edinburgh University and signatory of the American Declaration of Independence, had at one time accepted Mead's order of priorities, but experience of yellow fever persuaded him to reject the concept of contagion and advance the supremacy of local miasms.[11]

In Britain most of the medical community learned of this swing away from contagionism only at second hand, but the new epidemiology did gain some converts who made up for their small numbers by their propagandising. Leading their campaign against the quarantine system in the early 1820s was Charles Maclean, who had witnessed cholera in India and plague in the Levant (where to his temporary intellectual confusion he had caught the disease in a pest house). Through his efforts a parliamentary select committee sat in 1819 to evaluate plague's contagiousness and he later played a prominent role in the attempt to abolish quarantine regulations in Britain.[12] But on both occasions the prevailing orthodoxy retained control. A government commission on the cholera epidemic in Mauritius in 1819 unanimously concluded that 'the disease was contagious and was imported into Mauritius'.[13] The select committee on plague found that only two of the nineteen medical witnesses denied the disease's contagiousness. Their report concluded that 'If the committee had extended their examination to the whole of the faculty of London . . . they could not have raised more than one recruit for Dr Maclean . . .'[14]

Maclean's failure to influence Parliament in 1824–5 and his

death shortly before the new Quarantine Bill became law, reduced the anticontagionist propaganda for several years, although Thomas Southwood Smith, Physician to the London Fever Hospital, continued to be influenced by Maclean's ideas.[15] Smith, later to become notorious as Edwin Chadwick's sole medical colleague on the General Board of Health of 1848–53, held very firm and contentious views of disease causation in the 1820s, opinions which were to remain fixed and unyielding throughout his period of influence on official policy with Chadwick. Very broadly, Smith rejected the theories of atmospheric causation and contagion, asserting instead the primacy of local causes. 'As far as is yet known', he wrote in 1832, 'the exciting cause of all epidemic diseases is one and the same; namely a poison formed by the decomposition of organic matter. Vegetable and animal matter, during the process of putrefaction, give off a principal, or give origin to a new compound, which, when applied to the human body, produces the phenomena constituting fever.'[16] Although his unitary view of disease causation was to receive widespread condemnation in the medical press following the publication of his *Treatise on Fever* in 1830, Smith's rejection of contagion had gained considerable support after the 1828 yellow fever epidemic in Gibraltar, when a majority of the resident doctors and of the government's inspecting commission settled in favour of yellow fever's noncontagiousness.[17] Pym, president of the commission, was a predictable exception, as was, significantly, David Barry.[18] Cholera thus became a major issue in British medical circles at a time when controversy over disease causation already existed. The new disease became yet another pawn in a complex game between adherents of radically different philosophies.

The medical community began to polarise into two camps. To distinguish them as contagionists and noncontagionists is convenient but somewhat misleading, for neither group represented a systematic body of medical doctrine. Neither camp could claim to be unanimous over the respective merits of particular therapies, for example, nor was there necessarily any agreement over possible predisposing causes (x-factors). What did hold these amorphous groups together when discussing cholera was a common attitude to the quarantine system and, therefore, a common attitude to cholera's contagious properties.

Argument was to revolve around where cholera was to be placed on a spectrum of diseases which stretched from very contagious diseases at one pole to those which were totally uninfluenced by the contagious principle at the other. Unlike Smith, who was loath to admit any influence to contagionism, especially with the fevers and what Margaret Pelling has called 'the doubtful diseases', most medical men, or at least those who adhered to the concept of disease specificity, had their own views on which part of the spectrum to place each individual disease. Thus, while it is clear that it is too simplistic to divide the medical community simply into contagionists and noncontagionists, it is still useful to use these phrases when cholera alone is discussed, if only to show that medical men tended towards one or other end of the disease spectrum with this particular disease.

In 1831 contagionism was still dominant, the result of Britain's freedom from serious outbreaks of epidemic disease in the previous century. Whole generations of medical men had practised medicine whose only experience of epidemic disease came from increasingly out-of-date textbooks. Without the stimulus of frequent epidemics from abroad, epidemiology could not progress beyond its seventeenth-century position. Any medical opinion which opposed the contagionist viewpoint came up against one insuperable problem: the quarantine system was never tested (or at least it had never manifestly failed); therefore it could not be discredited.

Contagionism was also dominant because it was the official ideology of the Royal College of Physicians. While the Fellows' standpoint could be explained by reference to Britain's freedom from imported disease, also relevant was their common background of learning. Almost without exception they were products of the antediluvian system of medical education at Oxford and Cambridge, where in the eighteenth century medicine had ossified. Not until 1829 were some reforms, of a limited and ineffectual nature, introduced into the curriculum which took any account of the new developments in pathology, chemistry and physiology. Undue emphasis was still placed on the value of a literary education and a respect for ancient authority.[19]

But to claim that contagionism was merely the stronghold of conservatism and outmoded opinion would be to miss an essential point. It was a theory which could equally well be held by radicals and medical scientists well-versed in modern empirical techniques. Thomas Wakley was an obvious example of an ultra-radical professing contagionist principles (he was still a member of the National Union of the Working Classes in 1831). He decided in November 1831 that

> We can only suppose the existence of a poison which progresses independently of the wind, of the soil, of all conditions of the air, and of the barrier of the sea; in short, *one that makes mankind* the chief agent for its dissemination.[20]

The anomalous situation thus arose of Wakley siding with the anti-medical reformer, Roderick Macleod.[21]

An example of a physician aware of modern developments who could still be in the contagionist camp was David Barry. After spending his early career in the army, Barry received his M.D. from Edinburgh University in 1820. Between 1822 and 1827 he studied in Paris, where he carried out experiments on live dogs. One reviewer said of his subsequent research publication that it entitled Barry 'to a very high rank among the ablest physiologists of the present day'.[22] Barry was a contagionist because he believed that diseases could be transmitted by man, and possibly by goods also. This was the issue relating to cholera which clearly delineated the two opposing medical groups in London in 1831.

Contagionism, with quarantine, was an issue which touched on many sensitive areas. It was obviously to the country's economic interest that the medical community should reach some consensus but, given the prevailing attitudes of the time and the methods of analysis then available, this was an impossibility. The British medical profession was renowned for its ability to make accurate diagnoses, but success had always depended on the existence of evidence on which an acceptable theoretical structure could be built. It was not so much that evidence was lacking in 1831; rather, it was its contradictory nature which created difficulties. Originally, it was thought that British medical practitioners would have an advantage over their European counterparts because of the experience of the East India Company medical men. The Indian views had become known in Britain with the publication of the semi-official cholera reports from

Madras, Bengal and Bombay. While not generally available in Britain, they had been extensively reviewed in the medical press in the 1820s and two of them had been sent to the 'most eminent' of the profession in 1824. Other, smaller works, were printed in the medical journals during the same decade and in the summer of 1831 yet more tracts and monographs on cholera saturated the market. It was generally believed that most of the Indian works rejected contagionist ideas, but there were significant and important exceptions. The editor of the *Edinburgh Medical and Surgical Journal* found it comparatively easy to confirm his contagionist preconceptions from the Indian reports, while W. F. Chambers, lecturing on cholera at St George's Hospital London in February 1832, could inform his audience that the Madras Report was 'one of the great authorities referred to by the contagionists for materials to corroborate their notions of the novelty and progression of this pestilence.'[23]

Indeed, during the summer and autumn of 1831 more Indian doctors came out on the contagionist side. The first was James Kennedy, whose work on cholera became available in Britain at this time. William Russell returned from Russia with his noncontagionist opinions modified. Reginald Orton, who had opposed the contagionist 1819 Bombay Report, had been converted by the time the second edition of his book was published in London in 1831. 'The march of events,' he wrote, 'the great accumulation of facts and the gradual removal of prejudices, have wrought in my mind the same revolution they have in many others: the opinion of the contagious nature of the disease has been gradually gaining ground even in India, and seems to be the general one in Europe.'[24] All three men were respected for their knowledge of cholera.

Their changing attitudes, although comparatively rare at a time when opinions were hardening, reflected the basic weakness of medical science. Two factors, a set of contradictory data and an inadequate analytical methodology, ensured that discussions on cholera became inchoate, petty and increasingly shrill. Too many medical men were thinking in formal scholastic terms, relying on elaborate chains of reasoning, the evidence for which was random. Data which could not be fitted into the theory were discarded. Even the contagionist *London Medical Gazette* admitted that Kennedy's work, generally believed to be the best of its kind, had not included all the available data.[25] But to castigate the profession for sloppy and faulty reasoning would be unfair, for there was in 1831 no theory which enabled them to give an acceptable relative weighting to each piece of evidence. In Thomas Kuhn's parlance, medical science was still in a pre-paradigm period, in which all evidence appeared to be equally relevant.[26] Without a paradigm, which would have permitted the medical community to argue from a common starting point, the cholera debates were mutually contradictory. Rosen has rightly commented that

> Medical practice would be impossible without theories. Medical theory is not an adventure of the mind in the abstract, but an attempt at solving concrete, material problems. The factual knowledge essential to the physician in combating sickness would be of little use to him were it not for the theories which hold it together, systematize it, and give it meaning.[27]

The debates on cholera held at the London medical societies in 1831–2 demonstrated the prevailing mood of anarchy. The combatants could not even agree on the basic question of whether cholera was a specific disease, one school of thought, following Southwood Smith, arguing that there was only one disease which manifested itself with different symptoms according to the way local causes and the atmosphere reacted on each other. Once the evidence was assessed, it became clear that totally contradictory conclusions could be obtained from the data. To give but one example of many: one of the laws of contagious diseases was that doctors and nurses were more at risk than any other group because of their proximity to the sick. The evidence available could neither disprove nor sustain this theory, because when it was shown that in some places a disproportionate number of medical attendants were infected, noncontagionists were able to argue that this was proof of local miasms at work. Deadlock followed; mere guesses, of varying ingenuity, supplanted scientific theories.

Many practitioners were aware of their methodological inadequacies. Wakley, for example, believed that

> The progress of medicine, as an inductive science, is retarded by the construction of hypothetical theories, or the assumption of principles which are altogether gratuitous and imaginary,

and also by the deduction of general principles or conclusions, from a limited number of facts.[28]

P. H. Green argued that calm and ordered reflection was a prerequisite for scientific advancement,[29] but in the autumn of 1831 time was of the essence. The members of the community, whether of the old or new school, had perforce to rely almost exclusively on their powers of observation. The old school, epitomised by Halford, diagnosed purely by observing a patient's condition. It was still far from common for a doctor to check either the pulse or the temperature of a patient. Halford's was the Hippocratic method, which relied entirely on the physician's own sensations. The newer empirical school took diagnostics a stage further, by using the new sciences of pathology and physiology to correlate postmortem and clinical observations. It used the newest techniques during the heyday of morbid anatomy when autopsy was unfortunately still the only definitive diagnostic exercise.

Neither school of thought was, however, effective when there were no patients to examine. Reasoning by analogy was the only alternative, which ensured that confusions abounded, for much depended on which disease cholera was matched with. Contagionists, like Macmichael, compared cholera with the highly infectious smallpox, while noncontagionists theorised from the examples of the fevers, which they asserted were of local origin. The debates understandably made little headway and, given the circumstances in the autumn of 1831, the status quo remained unaltered. At the Westminster Medical Society in November Roderick Macleod argued that thirty-eight of forty medical men were contagionist, opting for what they regarded as the safest position. It is not very surprising that in the same month the noncontagionist *London Medical and Surgical Journal* claimed a great victory for the noncontagionists at the Westminster Medical Society.[30] For in addition to the weaknesses of available data and the prevailing method of arguing by analogy, the medical profession suffered from a limited and confusing terminology. It was not possible in 1831 to find an acceptable definition of the word contagion, even within the contagionist camp. Some continued to adhere to the strict contagionist position that a 'poison' was generated in the sick which could be transmitted, either by touch or breath, to the healthy. They came to use the words 'contagious' and 'infectious' indiscriminately. Macmichael, for example, following Mead's model, used the words synonymously in his essay on cholera.[31] Others, however, used the words more carefully. Indeed, Barry argued that the word contagion should be dropped completely. Experiments had led him to believe that a sick person exhuded a poison which penetrated the healthy through the lungs. All diseases were, therefore, infectious.[32] As he refused to accept that diseases could be spread by touch, contagion was useless as a distinguishing concept.

Barry's position demonstrates how in certain circumstances there was little difference between the theories put forward by both camps. By concentrating on a poison which travelled through the air from person to person, Barry was close to the ideas of Southwood Smith, who also believed that in rare instances and in very confined spaces the sick could generate a poison which the healthy could inhale. But what kept them apart was their different attitudes to quarantine, to disease specificity and to the doubtful diseases. Barry, before going to Russia, believed that a disease could be brought into a country both by men and goods. Yet this theoretical position was in fact modified by his experiences in Russia. Russell and Barry slowly came to agree that cholera was no more contagious than typhus, which many people, although not Southwood Smith and the extreme noncontagionists, accepted was the least contagious of all indigenous diseases. Goods could no longer, it was felt, harbour the disease. Russell and Barry's change of position was to have repercussions not only on government policy but also on the contagionist debate, which now moved to new ground where a consensus became more likely. Moreover, by the end of November 1831, with cholera confirmed in Britain, the question of quarantine had become academic; cholera's means of spread became the vital issue.

Unfortunately, because of the semantic confusions of the time, the somewhat closer theoretical position between the opposing groups was not fully appreciated. The situation became so involved at the Westminster Medical Society that

> there was a great confusion in the appreciation of the term contagion and infection. It is right to state the signification of these terms. *Contagion* is said to be a poison thrown off in the form of exhalation by putrefying animal and vegetable sub-

> stances, which is diffused through the air, and infects with disease the bodies of men and animals. *Infection* is the actual contamination of a healthy body by the morbid effluvia or exhalation, or contagion. Others have reversed the matter, use the words synonymously. Others again apply the term infection to that cause, whatever it may be which engenders endemic or epidemic diseases, and contagion the contamination of the system, either by inspiration of air into the lungs, by handling the sick, or by contact.[33]

But in reality the air was beginning to clear, primarily because the outbreak of cholera in Sunderland reduced the importance of the quarantine debate, ensured that Halford's extremist ultra-contagionist position was discredited as a significant help to the understanding of cholera, and enabled physicians personally to observe the disease. A change of mood can be detected and the theory of 'contingent contagionism' came into vogue.

Contingent contagionism was the position Russell and Barry were moving towards, but credit for publicising this theory, at least among the London physicians, must go to James Johnson. Born in Ireland in 1777, Johnson had served his apprenticeship with a surgeon-apothecary in County Antrim. During the Napoleonic Wars he served as surgeon's mate on various ships, being present in India during a cholera epidemic in 1804. In 1814 he treated the Duke of Clarence on HMS *Impregnable* and was rewarded with promotion to Surgeon-in-Ordinary. In 1816 Johnson began the *Medico-Chirurgical Review*, of which he was still editor in 1831. In 1821 he obtained his M.D. from Aberdeen University and became a licentiate of the Royal College of Physicians. His published works included the highly regarded *Influence of Tropical Climates on European Constitutions* (1812). 'In religion, general politics, and medical politics, Dr Johnson was known to be liberal, though free from scepticism, or ultra-radicalism.'[34]

Moderate in politics, Johnson was also moderate in his view of cholera. It was his intervention which had quelled cholera-phobia in June 1831. Confident that the British climate and social conditions would draw cholera's teeth (like most of the middle classes he seemed to be unaware of the plight of the poor), Johnson preached a doctrine which employed all three theories of disease causation then in use. He argued that 'In epidemic cholera, as in most other epidemics, a poison or sedative principle, whether emanating from the earth, from animal or vegetable bodies on the earth, or engendered in the air, strikes a predisposed individual, and after an uncertain period of incubation, produces a state of phenomena.' In accepting that the proximate cause of cholera was a chemical reaction occurring through the agency of the air or of rotting vegetable matter, Johnson was no different from Southwood Smith, but he also believed that in certain circumstances, especially low-lying and filthy surroundings, cholera could be communicated from person to person. He thus accentuated the malarial and aerial principles together with their possible infectious nature. He also laid particular emphasis on what he called 'contingencies', circumstances, *not humours*, which predisposed certain people to suffer disease. For typhus, the contingencies were overcrowding and filthy conditions. Remove them and the infectious principle was destroyed. By the use of analogy, Johnson suggested that the same contingencies applied to cholera, especially after Russell and Barry reported that cholera was no more infectious than typhus. Ensure cleanliness and ventilation and the infectious character of cholera would be destroyed.[35]

Johnson was, of course, by no stretch of the imagination an original thinker. Like Barry he bridged the divide between the contagionists and their extreme opponents; his importance lay in the all-embracing nature of his proposals, his stress on environmental predisposing causes and the esteem with which he was held by the medical profession. He had put forward a synthesis of existing theories which gave his colleagues an opportunity of ending the fruitless quarrels over fundamentals. Contingent contagionism gave an escape route to those extreme contagionists, who were beginning to lose confidence, along which they could retreat without totally losing prestige.

By stressing environmental predisposing causes, it also helped to synthesize the data which came from the North-East. Cholera had spread only slowly, in accordance with the principles of contagious diseases. 'It crept, like a skulking hyena, from one dirty lane to another, seizing those who were half in the grave already, or who, from terror, were flying before the enemy.'[36] Those who witnessed such happenings in the North-East, both visiting doctors and local men such as E. H. Greenhow, who was later to be prominent in the public health movement, did not now have to become confirmed contagionists or even agnostics; a suitable theory existed which took all the variables into account. Above all environmental predisposing causes explained why some people caught a disease and others did not. Those who suffered did so as a result of some deficiency in their lifestyles. It was obviously a concept which appealed to the moralistic side of the profession. Many agreed that 'Intemperance gives a claim to the pestilence which it never overlooks; in every town and district, from the Ganges to the Wear, the drunkard has been the object of its earliest attack and its most ruthless visitation.'[37] The idea received a boost from the spectacular cholera outbreak in Gateshead during the Christmas celebrations and was to explain why the disease was frequently at its worst following the weekend bout of drinking.

An irregular diet was also seen as a predisposing cause. Indian doctors had considered it so since Dr Tytler had attributed the 1817 cholera outbreak in Jessore to blighted rice.[38] In Britain, due partly to the confusion between English and Asiastic cholera, soft fruit and vegetables were considered possible predisposing causes. The Central Board of Health even suggested 'the maintenance of a moderately constipated state of the bowels as an important preservative during the prevalence of the epidemic'.[39] Excessive eating helped to explain why some of the better classes caught the disease. Craigie, for example, believed that the vicar of Newburn died because of eating pickled salmon. It better suited his noncontagionist views to explain the vicar's death in this manner than to accept that the disease had been relayed during visits to the sick (though even this explanation could have been fitted into less extreme noncontagionist theory). Commonsense in the light of the usual crop of bowel complaints during the summer, suggested that eating habits should be rigorously checked. And when, as in Manchester, potatoes which had been vomited emitted a phosphorescent light for several days, one wonders why any other explanation should henceforward have been sought![40]

The concept of environmental predisposing causes was the new x-factor in the theoretical equation. But, unlike those of earlier years, it was not metaphysical but deeply rooted in social realities. Predisposing causes were tangible and led to social prophylaxis. The concept was doubly important to the medical profession because it allowed them to bypass their main role as curers of disease, and turn to promoting measures which were feasible and which offered the opportunity of preventing epidemic disease. Preventive medicine became a major objective for many in the profession, including J. P. Kay in Manchester, Robert Baker in Leeds and James Lawrie in Scotland. In the drive for public health reform the medical community, or rather a significant number of individual doctors, were to play a major role. Without the contingent contagionist theory it is doubtful whether so many would have been active. The theory acted as a half-way house for many who, while finding the old contagionist position no longer tenable, could still not accept the full miasmatist theory. It therefore carried along the same path as Edwin Chadwick many who found the equation dirt—disease too simplistic. By the end of 1831 it influenced the editors both of the *Edinburgh Medical and Surgical Journal* and *The Lancet* and there is some reason for supposing that Roderick Macleod saw the light.

If contingent contagionism was to have major long-term consequences (it included among its adherents Sir John Simon and was to survive as an intellectual force until the end of the century),[41] David Barry at the Central Board of Health ensured that it was influential in 1832. The precautionary measures suggested by the Board were consistent with the contingent contagionist position. When the Board came to analyse the reports which some of the local boards drew up after the epidemic, the varying evidence could only be synthesized by reference to contingent contagionism. Although still preferring to stress the importance of paupers and vagrants in spreading cholera, the Central Board admitted that pure contagionism was not the only theory capable of explaining the disease's puzzling mode of transmission.[42] In 1832, therefore, contingent contagionism became official orthodoxy.

As a paradigm, however, capable of uniting all of the medical profession behind an all-embracing ideology, contingent contagionism eventually failed in 1832. Like Chartism later, it spread its net too wide. As the disease spread from the North-East, medical men witnessing it for the first time theorised only from their own personal observations. Cholera's appearance in London resurrected the hoary question of its long-distance transmission. Debates in the medical societies became ever more vigorous and vituperative, until at the final session of the Westminster Medical Society A. Bozzi Granville insisted that a vote be taken on cholera's contagiousness. Although against the society's rules a vote was taken which went in favour of the noncontagionists, but only by twenty-four votes to twenty-two. As James Greenwood complained, many contagionists had failed to attend the meeting; otherwise the decision would have been reversed.[43]

Six months of debate had therefore ended inconclusively with factionalism rampant. Thereafter no genuine attempt was made to verify observations or compare them with the experiences of others. The conceptual apparatus capable of dealing with very complex issues was lacking. As Winslow has noted, 'Until the theory of inanimate contagion was replaced by a theory of living germs and until to that theory were added the concepts of long-distance transmission by water and food supplies and, above all, of human and animal carriers, the hypothesis of contagion would not work.'[44] It is true that all these ideas were raised in Britain in 1832. Several writers suggested that cholera was caused by tiny animaculae invisible to the naked eye. Not being capable of proof, their views were rightly taken no more seriously than any other 'eccentric' theory put forward. Neither was water regarded as a possible medium for cholera's transmission, for all the doctrines from the past had stressed the importance of the atmosphere. The possibilities for explanation of disease causation were far greater when more observable factors such as filth and nuisances were examined. They, it should be stressed, were seen as possible seats of the poison and not as vectors. Finally, a crude form of carrier concept was suggested in 1831–2, mainly by contagionists.[45] William Russell hinted at the possibility but failed to draw any conclusions.

> It seems tolerably well ascertained that the cholera has not broken out spontaneously in any place without communication by persons or effects coming from infected places; but it is somewhat singular and unaccountable that the disease has appeared in situations where the persons arriving did not themselves labour under the disease at the time of their arrival.[46]

Roderick Macleod was quick to point out that such a theory would help to explain the difficulties involved in tracing the linkages between the infected,[47] but of course there was no way of proving this without a knowledge of micro-organisms and of the role water played as a medium.

Given the contradictory data, the methods of reasoning and the confusions of terminology, it is not surprising that the medical profession tied itself in knots in 1832. Without a body of pure research scientists available to set minimum standards, each theory put forward, and there were literally hundreds, appeared as attractive or as ineffectual as the next; dogmatism and nihilism resulted. The medical community was as widely divided at the end of 1832 as it had been in the autumn of 1831, although it is probably true to say that contingent contagionism had penetrated to a considerable extent. The antics which the profession underwent contrasts curiously with the virtual unanimity displayed by its counterpart in the United States. According to Rosenberg, 'A sample of the opinions expressed by 109 American physicians during the years 1832–34 shows that ninety did not consider the disease to be at all contagious, while only five considered the disease to be primarily contagious. The other fourteen considered it to be primarily noncontagious but admitted that under some circumstances cholera might become communicable (contingent contagionism).'[48] An explanation for this contrast can be seen by referring to the epidemiological histories of the two countries. Britain in 1832 was undergoing the same scientific stage as the United States had passed through during the yellow fever epidemics in the 1790s. The defeat of pure contagionism had occurred forty years earlier in the New World when the old orthodoxy, tainted by colonialism, was overthrown by Rush and other patriots. In Britain, however, the eighteenth-century structure of the medical profession, and with it its dominant ideology, remained intact, if somewhat bloodied, in 1831. What, during the cholera years, was regarded as orthodoxy in the United States, was seen to be heresy in Britain. By 1848, with Chadwick and Southwood Smith representing official doctrine, circumstances seem to have changed dramatically. But as shall be shown later, such an apparent *volte face* by the British medical profession masks considerable support for, if not pure contagionism, at least contingent contagionism.

The debates on the nature of the new disease were, therefore, inconclusive in 1831–2, but they did make clear that, in the absence of convincing information, many medical practitioners preferred to opt for the safest position, that of some variant of contagionism. This safety-first policy can be seen to be the dominant position taken by the medical community in all its dealings with cholera in 1832, especially when it came to therapy. To understand fully the reasons for this, it is necessary to revert to the Orders in Council issued in preparation for the epidemic.

If the appearance of cholera had diminished the influence of the elitist Royal College of Physicians in government circles, it had raised the position of the lower echelons of the medical community in the provinces. The Order in Council of October 1831 had recommended the establishment of local boards of health, membership to consist of some magistrates, the clergy, two or more medical men and three or more of the principal inhabitants. Possibly for the first time, most members of the medical community were given some official recognition and placed hierarchically in close conjunction with the elite groups in local society. The significance of this was not fully recognised at the time. Wakley, for instance, was indignant that local medical men were not given a more important role to play. The regulations, he wrote, should be 'looked upon as little short of premeditated deliberate insult, offered to a majority of general practitioners' by the Royal College of Physicians.[49] Every medical man, he continued, should be on the board, and they should have the entire control of public health measures.

Wakley failed to perceive how the local boards were to work in practice. In the smaller communities, and especially in the rural areas, two medical men may well have been the sum total of qualified practitioners available for selection to the board. In the larger towns, the local boards were recommended to establish sub-district boards, on which medical men also served. While the system certainly did not place all practitioners on the same social footing, it did encourage interplay between the different status groups. In York, for instance, the Central Committee included all the city's physicians and the six senior surgeons, who combined to become a General Medical Board. Under their direction the rest of the medical community worked on the parish committees with the clergy, overseers and principal inhabitants. The local board structure, while confirming the internal hierarchy of the medical community, helped to raise the status of the apothecary and general practitioner *at the parish level.*

Many practitioners must have found themselves basking in newly-found and unexpected popularity during the period before cholera arrived. But the appearance of the disease on British soil was to cause considerable difficulties. In some places, most especially in the North-East of England, the medical community as a whole was to find that its medical opinions had to be altered to suit the convenience of the local ruling elites, who wanted scientific confirmation of their claim that cholera was not an imported disease. But for most practitioners throughout the country the most pressing problem was how to treat the disease. On the results of their therapy depended their future prestige, both collectively and individually.

Any attempt to evaluate the treatments administered to cholera victims in 1832 must be preceded by some assessment of the drugs available for use. It should be stressed that specific remedies were extremely rare at this time. Most drugs available were merely palliative, at best diminishing the side-effects of a disease without affecting the particular micro-organism at work. Some new drugs, such as morphine, quinine and, in 1832, codeine had been isolated, but they had not been fully tested, nor had they been included in the most recent pharmacopoeia. Indeed, one London medical journal commented in 1832, 'It is passing strange that our *Pharmacopoeia* should always be behind the progress of science.'[50] While it was probably advantageous to the sick that such new and toxic drugs as prussic acid failed to be included in pharmacopoeias even fifty years after discovery, the lack of choice in therapy open to the medical community ensured that in 1832 they came to rely heavily on traditional remedies.

One of the most common treatments in 1832 was bloodletting, which was administered for a variety of conditions, but primarily as a means of reducing inflammation in certain types of fever and pneumonia.[51] This practice had been the subject of much debate in the previous twenty years, between those practitioners who believed fevers to be characterised by debility (which contra-indicated bloodletting) and those who, like Henry Clutterbuck and John Armstrong, felt them to be inflammatory and therefore recommended copious and immediate bloodletting to reduce congestion. Before Clutterbuck and Armstrong's 'bloodletting revolution', medical opinion, influenced by a realisation that urban fevers were increasingly a function of the debilitating effects of deficient nutrition, eschewed the practice. But gradually, as the belief that fevers were not the consequence of indigence gained influence, Clutterbuck could claim in 1819 that, 'A great revolution is taking place in the treatment of this disease. Bloodletting, which, but a few years ago, was looked upon with abhorrence in the cure of contagious fever . . . is proved, by ample testimony, to be not only the most powerful, but the safest of remedies . . .'.[52]

The practice of venesection in fevers was dependent on the clinical decisions made by each individual practitioner, although those who were moving towards a unitary view of fever in the 1820s especially emphasised its importance. Likewise, in 1832, its practice on cholera victims was dependent partly on whether the practitioner felt the disease to be inflammatory or debilitating, although even for the traditionalists the presence of copious evacuations in cholera cases suggested the disease to be inflammatory and suitable for bloodletting. Understandably, therefore, practitioners of all persuasions could justify bloodletting and the practice was extensively indulged in, usually as the first preliminary step in a long course of treatment.

One historian has been particularly critical of those who practised venesection on cholera victims.

> No more harmful medical intervention could be conceived than the removal of already depleted blood. Yet for many years bleeding was the standard treatment for cholera. Tens of thousands of cholera patients must have been despatched by their physicians to their graves, much as the kosher butcher slaughters his victims.[53]

Howard-Jones' article considers cholera therapy in Europe throughout the nineteenth century, but with reference to venesection he is concerned only with the first pandemic, for he states that the practice had fallen out of fashion by 1848. He seems to make two assertions: one is the obvious accusation of mass killing; the other, more insidious, is the implication that the *motives* of medical practitioners were suspect. His analogy suggests the ritual slaughter by those whom he called benevolently homicidal. Before whose altar the victims were sacrificed and for what mystic reason we are left to surmise. Before considering Howard-Jones' assertion in detail, it will be useful to examine modern medical opinion on bloodletting.[54] The blood volume of healthy people averages five litres. The removal of one pint (*c.* 460ml.) from a healthy person may cause a little faintness but generally causes no symptoms which persist for longer than thirty minutes. A sudden loss of two pints of blood, amounting to 20 per cent of the total circulating blood volume, causes faintness and some shock with elevation of the pulse rate and fall in the blood pressure. A sudden loss of anything more than one and a half litres, about 30 per cent of circulating blood volume, could give rise to profound shock and possibly death.

In severe cases of cholera the erythrocyte count may rise as high as eight or nine million cells/cubic mm, indicating a loss of at least half of the plasma volume and perhaps 25 per cent of circulating blood volume. Death would result from this loss of blood volume, and also from the haemoconcentration and increase in blood viscosity (i.e. what doctors in 1832 referred to as the 'tarry' nature of the blood). It is clear that in this situation bloodletting would very likely be fatal.

Venesection, therefore, neither cured a patient, nor alleviated the symptoms of cholera. But the *degree* of harm inflicted depended on two factors: the volume of blood removed by the doctor; and the stage of the disease at which depletion took place. A token depletion of twenty to thirty ml would have no impact on the course of the disease. Much more than that and the treatment would actually aid *V. cholerae* more than the patient. It is, of course, impossible to determine the volume of blood removed by medical men in 1832, although we can assume that in general more blood would be removed by using the lancet than by cupping, and more by cupping than by leeches. However, some indication of the possible harm being inflicted can be gauged from knowledge of when bloodletting took place, and what its purpose was. Having examined most of the cases of cholera treatment reported in the medical journals in 1832, it is clear that venesection was practised most frequently when a doctor *first saw* his patient. While motives for its use at this stage varied, it was frequently believed to relieve congestion by turning the circulation of the blood from the centre to the surface of the body. If the success of this practice was measured by an increase in the pulse rate, then it suggests that doctors were removing less than 20 per cent of the circulating blood volume. The impulse to remove a huge volume of blood, which would have been in keeping with Armstrong's precepts, seems to have been kept in check in 1832, possibly because the bloodletting revolution had begun to fizzle out by the end of the 1820s.[55] In most cases, therefore, we should view venesection as a reflex action on the part of the physician as soon as he entered a sick room, in much the same way as a modern general practitioner automatically reaches for his thermometer. It was the essential preliminary action, clearing the way for a reasoned diagnosis to be made.

Pragmatic considerations also prevented venesection being practised at a later stage of the disease, for as the electrolytes and water were voided from the victim, blood became almost impossible to obtain. Howard-Jones claims that some medical men attempted venesection at all stages of the disease, but he fails to appreciate that they were in a minority and, moreover, had developed this practice *in India*; there is little evidence to suggest that this was a widespread habit in Britain in 1832.

It follows from the above that if venesection was a fatal procedure on its own, then it should have been reflected in the number of persons dying from cholera at an early stage. But to my knowledge there is no evidence of this happening on any significant scale. It is true that, particularly when cholera first infected a community, deaths sometimes occurred within a remarkably short period of time. Of the first five confirmed deaths from cholera in London, for example, one died within eight hours of onset and three others within fifteen hours. But this seems to have been a consequence of the disease whether or not venesection had been practised: a swift death, therefore, was not a consequence of the therapy applied.

Unfortunately, there is very little data giving a breakdown of periods of sickness before death in this epidemic. Isolated examples, given as evidence of the horrors of cholera in the newspapers and medical journals, obviously prove the case neither one way nor the other. But there is some very revealing evidence from Exeter. Thomas Shapter accumulated data on the duration of attack of 335 of the 402 deaths in that city (see Table 5.1).

Table 5.1. Duration of Illness Before Death from Cholera in Exeter, 1832

	Hours				Days					
	Under 6	6-11	12-17	18-24	1-2	2-3	3-4	4-5	5-6	6+
Males	2	7	9	49	53	17	7	6	5	11
Females	0	10	5	51	57	15	5	3	6	17

Source: T. Shapter, *History of Cholera in Exeter in 1832*, p 219.

Assuming that anyone dying after twelve hours from onset went through all three stages of the disease, only 5.6 per cent of the 335 victims *may* have succumbed to the physician's lancet. If the assumption is made that the periods of sickness of the other sixty-seven victims were not recorded because they were not treated by a doctor, and that therefore they could not have been victims of treatment, only 4.7 per cent of total deaths may possibly have resulted from the activities of the local medical profession.

Such evidence does not exonerate the medical community from on occasion helping the demise of a patient, but it certainly suggests that accusations of mass killing must be regarded as pure hyperbole. However, in order to probe the motives of practitioners, let us assume that bloodletting was a fatal exercise. Why should medical men pursue a therapy which was manifestly killing more than it cured? Were they automatons blindly following their theoretical preconceptions, even though the therapy was contra-indicated? This was obviously not the case. Bloodletting was common because of the *observed* fact that while it did not cure, neither did it harm.[56] Moreover, one pertinent reason for the practitioners' belief in bloodletting's harmlessness was the frequency with which they were treating other than true cholera victims, usually those suffering from either choleraeic diarrhoea, cholerine or even the common summer diarrhoea. When this fact is combined with the knowledge that the local authorities unwittingly encouraged those suffering from mild forms of disease to visit a practitioner by exhorting everyone with any form of bowel disorder to seek immediate medical help, it is not surprising that venesection seemed harmless.

Similar considerations are equally relevant in explaining the repeated use of calomel and opium, the traditional English therapy developed in India. Either on its own or in conjunction with opium, calomel was the most frequently used drug in Britain in 1832, being recommended by the Central Board of Health in London. Howard-Jones' treatment of this therapy is both brief and hostile; he is content to emphasise the enormous quantities of calomel being proposed by the Hull physician Joseph Ayres in the middle of the century.[57] But the implication that Ayres, with his enormous dosages, was typical of medical men at this time, is erroneous. In fact Ayres was very much in the minority, for he claimed his preparation of calomel to be a specific cure, not part of a plan of treatment aimed modestly (and realistically) at relieving symptoms.[58]

Calomel was used as a cathartic, but as a compound of mercury it is toxic. Understandably, it no longer figures in modern pharmacopoeias, although interestingly enough it remained in the historical section of Goodman and Gilman's *Pharmacological Basis of Therapeutics* until very recently. However, because calomel was replaced long ago, it is not now known how effective its cathartic properties were.[59]

To suggest that calomel saved lives on any significant scale would be altogether too sanguine, yet it is equally doubtful that it caused death. Even Joseph Ayres, with his massive doses of calomel, claimed an extremely high success rate, although this should be treated with some caution.

In the same way as venesection was legitimised by its apparent beneficial effect on the pulse rate, calomel could also be justified on empirical grounds, for the appearance of green stools was regarded as a favourable sign, and calomel had this effect.[60]

Calomel was usually administered with opium or its compound laudanum. Opium acts as a constipator and analgesic but has no specific effect on *V. cholerae*. In 1832 many physicians were aware of the dangers stemming from its overuse. The most scathing criticism came from John Alderson, Ayre's rival in Hull.

> Mercury and opium have ever been . . . the sheet anchor of the quack; and on the first appearance of cholera . . . there was great disposition to employ them. . . . It appears at present that

> ample experience has brought the practice much into disrepute in cholera, and although calomel and opium still continue to be given in all doses, and at all intervals throughout the disease, there are few advocates found for their indiscriminate use.[61]

Embroiled in his controversy with Ayres, Alderson underestimated opium's popularity, for it had many advocates, some of whom prescribed vast quantities.[62]

Unfortunately, it has not been possible to obtain quantifiable data on case fatality rates for each major therapy to confirm the hypothesis that in 1832 medical intervention was not significantly destructive of life. What records have remained are very fragmentary and result in suspiciously low case fatality rates.[63] Indeed, no serious attempt was made to evaluate the effectiveness of different treatments until the third cholera epidemic in 1853–4. Apart from bloodletting, which had been discredited by the epidemic of 1848–9, the drugs administered in 1853 remained depressingly similar to 1832 even though some new therapies, such as sulphuric acid and ether, were administered without success in 1853. Following that epidemic, the Treatment Committee of the Medical Council issued a report on the value of major treatments, which can be used here effectively to offer some suggestions as to the relative safety of the treatments administered in 1832. Table 5.2 gives the case fatality rates of those drugs prescribed in 1853–4 which were commonly used in 1832, together, for comparison, with the rates of some of the more favoured newer therapies.

Although the fatality rates are frighteningly high from a modern perspective, they still suggest that practitioners in 1832 by and large did their best with the materials available. First, the drugs most frequently administered in 1832 were still in 1853–4, except for sulphuric acid, those offering the greatest 'success' rate. The number of remedies may have been few, but from a limited array most medical men chose wisely, except for those who continued to administer laxatives (and they were frequently criticised in 1832). The passing of a further thirty years had resulted in only one new therapy, sulphuric acid, which could compare with calomel, opium and the saline treatment for relative effectiveness.

But the crucial question has still to be answered: would fewer of these victims have died if they had not been subjected to the interventions of medicine? One reputable modern prognosis of untreated cholera cases states, 'As many as 50 per cent to 75 per cent of dehydrated cholera patients who are not appropriately treated die either from shock within the first day of illness or from secondary effects after a week or so.'[64] This suggests that medical intervention in the nineteenth century may have been

Table 5.2 Case Fatality Rates from Selected Remedies in London, 1853–54

Remedy	Cases	Deaths	Fatality Rate %
Calomel (small)	584	275	47
Calomel (large)	582	261	45
Calomel & opium	301	109	36
Salines	166	78	47
Castor Oil	124	89	72
Sulphuric Acid	408	191	47
Ether	28	23	82

Source: Report from the treatment committee of the Medical Council, PP, xlv, 1854–55, 4-11.

slightly effective, or at least not overly hazardous. John Simon was possibly being too pessimistic when he wrote in 1867, following what was to be the last cholera epidemic in Britain, that 'our utmost power is but perhaps some very little ability of palliation'.[65]

Many other remedies were administered in 1832, but those discussed above were by far the most common. Others, such as rhubarb, peppermint and ginger, were of purely cosmetic value, but some, croton oil and cauterisation for example, were certainly extremely harmful. But perhaps the one saving grace was their infrequent use, the fate of all new or original therapies in 1832, for it seems that cautious medical practitioners rejected new remedies following only a few failures. Intravenous saline injections are a good case in point.

Usually discussed totally separately from croton oil and cauterisation because it is now seen as the forerunner of a successful therapy, the history of intravenous saline infusion in 1832 should be seen as a paradigm of all newer drugs and techniques, for it too failed to give successful clinical results. The possibility of death from air embolism or septicaemia; the natural caution of its promoter William Brooke O'Shaughnessy, who advised its use only in terminal cases;[66] the difficulties involved in performing the operation—all coincided to ensure failure.

Thus, as with croton oil and cauterisation, intravenous saline infusion was discarded. But it is important to recognise that it was the same rigorous demand for empirical confirmation of theory which led to the demise of *both* potentially useful *and* potentially dangerous therapies. Nevertheless, the experimentation which did take place demonstrated that it was possible for early nineteenth-century medical men to observe a new disease, theorise on its effects, and then test the theories. A real scientific spirit was abroad in Britain. There was a receptiveness to new ideas, in whose diffusion the medical journals played a crucial role. Dr Thomas Latta first gave intravenous saline therapy a fillip by testing it with some initial success after reading of O'Shaughnessy's ideas in *The Lancet*.[67] The Central Board of Health in London also played a vital role, by passing on information to the medical journals. Sir David Barry, a member of the Board, personally requested several practitioners in the provinces to test O'Shaughnessy's proposals;[68] a willing and able audience was waiting for just such a lead. The fact that new ideas such as intravenous therapy could penetrate through to an isolated practitioner like John Langworthy in the rural parish of Plympton St Mary in Devon—and could then be tested—gives a new insight into the medical community in 1832.[69] Of course, opposition to the new ideas was frequently overwhelming, but this should not be regarded as obscurantist obstructionism. It was also a sign of medical science's growing professionalism; those who tested the new ideas were playing devil's advocate, in the same way as editors of medical and scientific journals were to later in the century, as they sifted the gold from the dross in research papers.

Traditional treatment was thus justified on solid, medical grounds, but it was reinforced by social and intra-professional pressures exerted on medical men at the same time. Any prolonged testing of a new therapy which failed to show successful clinical results endangered whatever social standing and respect the practitioner had attained. This applied whether he was a London physician, a member of an upwardly mobile group in the provinces, or an isolated practitioner in the countryside. There is no doubt that much could be gained by displaying, both collectively and individually, reasoned judgement and calmness at the bedside; in a period of crisis the relatives of a victim would be expecting reassurance and comfort from the medical man, not experimentation. It was certainly the case in Plympton St Mary that relatives of the sick awaited the arrival of Langworthy with tense anticipation.[70] Nor did he let them down. Almost dropping from fatigue, he rode across his vast practice doing what little he could to alleviate suffering. He was by no means a hick doctor; he read of intravenous saline infusions in *The Lancet* and tested them, but the need to visit other patients prevented him giving the system a fair trial. There is no doubt that Langworthy's exertions, and the help given by the local incumbent, gave a great psychological boost to both patients and relatives. Indeed, one does not know whether he assuaged fear and anxiety not just by being present, but precisely *because* he used traditional remedies. Janet Blackman has shown how long it might take for medical knowledge to percolate down the social scale and how it might be moulded to fit existing popular perceptions.[71] Bloodletting might well have been tolerable;[72] newer techniques, especially the external therapies such as cauterisation and the cold water treatment (the latter suggesting the treatment given to the insane), probably were not. Thus, by keeping to old and tested remedies, the medical community might have reinforced popular perceptions, reduced suspicion of official medicine and raised or at least confirmed the social position of the individual practitioner. Much could have been lost by a frivolous regard for innovation for its own sake.

Not every practitioner in 1832, however, preferred to pursue a safety-first policy. There were some who saw the epidemic as a means of promoting their own personal status, both within the medical and the local communities, by claiming to have discovered specific cures. A prime example of this was Dr William Stevens, who had first suggested his saline plan (the infusion orally and per rectum of a solution of neutral salts) to treat yellow fever patients in Tobago in the late 1820s.[73] Stevens can be seen as a prime example of those medical men who used a specific as a way to gain both fame and an entrance into the relatively closed world of the medical establishment. His treatment was at first taken extremely seriously and the Central Board of Health recommended its testing. But in June 1832 Stevens claimed the cure of ninety-two cholera victims in Cold Bath Fields House of Correction in London. A Central Board medical team found that none of the patients had been suffering from cholera; one was diagnosed as a suitable case for a dentist.[74] Stevens' reputation was destroyed; his actions gave some support to James Johnson's claim that he was mentally unstable.[75] The combination of unsuccessful clinical results and the social disgrace of its mentor ensured that the saline therapy was totally discredited, although variants of it were to be used in later epidemics.

Stevens had tried unsuccessfully to break into the citadel of official medicine in London. Another who found similar difficulties was Thomas Latta, when he promoted intravenous saline infusions in Edinburgh, the other major city firmly controlled by socially prestigious physicians. Latta had read of O'Shaughnessy's treatment in *The Lancet* and had tested it with occasional success in Edinburgh. His 'crime' of reporting his findings was condemned on two grounds: the therapy had developed from the new science of chemical pathology and was therefore regarded with suspicion by those clinging to older schools of thought; and Latta himself was outside the charmed circle of the Edinburgh medical establishment.[76] He was condemned by those who had the power and prestige to hinder the reception of new ideas. Again, the combination of dubious results and fear for the status quo within medicine influenced both opinion and action in 1832.

In the provinces, however, where official medicine was not so firmly entrenched, promoters of new therapies still found themselves involved in intra-professional disputes. Clashes occurred in Manchester and Liverpool,[77] but the most colourful occurred in Hull, and involved Dr Joseph Ayres, in which a challenge to a duel was issued, with the vanquished to quit town. That such unseemly disputes could harm the profession's reputation can be seen from the following verse, published in the radical James Acland's *Hull Portfolio*.

The Physicians of Hull,
Must of patients be null,
Thus to wage with each other dire war;
When they meet in divan
On some Choleric plan
And squabble, pull noses and spar.

When the matter to mend
Lest too soon it should end
And their valour not shine full before ye,
Each put out his tract
To state the true fact
And claim to the whole of the glory.

But one—(it is true)
Gets this done by his crew
Like a kind of secondhand bully;
So the worshipful clan
Fall foul of their man
Who deservedly bastes them, most fully.

And thus stands the matter
That makes a town's clatter,
For parties get higher and louder;
E'en the lads of 'the school'
Think the best way to cool,
A pestle, a pill and some powder.[78]

Ayres was the true culprit, a provincial practitioner seeking prestige by claiming a specific cure for cholera which was 'not merely successful, but eminently successful'.[79] His specific was not original, being merely vast quantities of calomel and opium, but, as shown above, it may have been *relatively* successful. Ayres was a persistent character and was to be found as late as the 1850s hawking his cures around the medical journals.[80]

It was one of Ayres' opponents, John Alderson, who most clearly pointed to the alternative approaches which a practitioner could take in 1832.

> On the appearance of any new disease there are always two objects, towards the attainment of which the efforts of the

medical world are directed. First, the discovery of a specific remedy; secondly, the establishment, by observation and comparison, of such just views of the pathology of the disease as may form the basis of a rational plan of treatment.[81]

Alderson was firmly in favour of the second objective; only those seeking 'easy public success' would ever claim to have discovered a specific cure for cholera.

Practitioners such as Stevens and Ayres were very much in a minority in 1832, most medical men preferring to follow Alderson in seeking a rational plan of treatment. But Ayres received much more national publicity than Alderson; as a result, historians have tended to accentuate the importance of the mavericks in the medical community and to neglect the majority who responded to cholera in a traditional and 'safe' manner.[82]

One result of this has been the failure to perceive that, for most of the medical community in 1832, the desire to relieve suffering, and the need to gain status both in the eyes of their peers and in lay society, usually dovetailed to encourage medical men to persist with tried and tested therapies. Most combated cholera manfully, with both compassion and fortitude.[83] Some died treating the sick; many suffered from overwork and overstrain, as did Langworthy in Devon and Daun in the North-East.[84] They have been unjustly maligned by one historian who claims their intervention 'often had disastrous consequences' and by another who feels that throughout the nineteenth century they overestimated the benefits they could offer.[85] The former criticism neglects to consider what alternatives were open in 1832, and what lay opinion on new therapy might have been; the latter overemphasises the thrusting attitude of one small section of the medical community. A practitioner of that era, like everyone else, was the product of his times and worked within the framework of contemporary ideas and realities. To expect greater results from early nineteenth-century medical science is to be anachronistic. As exemplars of their own era, practitioners reacted according to their own logic and value systems. It is salutary to remember that even today, faced with an incurable disease, medical science can only offer treatment for symptoms and try to reduce pain and suffering. Social and professional pressures coincided with the practical results of medical therapy in 1832 to ensure that caution and pragmatism epitomised medical action. The medical community as a whole was probably no more popular after the disease had disappeared, but individual medical men certainly came out of the epidemic with increased prestige and honour. By sticking to traditional modes of therapy and by eschewing reckless experimentation,[86] medical men confirmed their social position in 1832;[87] by not losing ground during this temporary crisis they were able to proceed with their aim of achieving personal and collective social 'comfort'.

6

Cholera and the Propertied Classes

It has already been pointed out that government response to the threat from cholera in 1831 was in part conditioned by knowledge of the widespread popular insurrections in Eastern Europe which followed in cholera's wake. In Britain the Swing riots in the agricultural south in 1830 and the first disturbances consequent to the movement for parliamentary reform in 1831 had shown that society, still unsettled by the long-term stresses which industrialisation imposed, was in a state of flux. Some unexpected and additional threat to the social order, it was feared, could spark off a general conflagration. For the propertied classes, those who controlled the community's economic, legal and social resources, cholera might be the final straw which broke the camel's back. Its recognised partiality for the poor and propertyless made it a suitable medium for highlighting the major inequalities and structural weaknesses of British society. The ways in which the propertied responded to this threat to the social order can illustrate their attitudes and relationships towards other social groups and their own conceptions of the state of society at a time of general unrest.

The British reading public first became aware of cholera when Russia was infected in 1830, but it was not until the disease reached the Baltic ports that they began actively to respond to the threat. The possibility of cholera's arrival in Britain precipitated a wave of general apprehension known as choleraphobia. Charles Greville noted on 19 June 1831 that news of Riga's infection

> . . . soon diffused a general alarm, and for many days past the newspapers have been full of letters and full of lies, and every sort of representation is made to Government or through the press, as fear or interest happens to dictate. . . . This topic

> has now occupied for some days a good deal of the attention even of the fine fools of this town.[1]

Choleraphobia was symptomatised by a spate of (false) cholera cases and accentuated by the unfortunate coincidence of the name of this new disease with the common or English cholera (i.e. summer diarrhoea), which was prevalent, but rarely fatal, in the summer months. Uncertainty surrounding cholera's symptomatology resulted in the publication even of fever cases as those of *Cholera Morbus*. Such was the alarm that for a few weeks cholera vied with political questions as the major talking point.

> This subject [cholera] divides attention with the Reform Bill. No medical man can enter a house without being questioned about it; and the papers, both at home and abroad, teem with the most alarming accounts. In short, there is complete panic; and as mankind are ever prone to magnify horrors, so we trust that the extent to which the disease has prevailed, as well as its rate of mortality, will be found to have been exaggerated.[2]

T. B. Macaulay wrote to his sister from London at this time, 'The great topic now . . . is not, as you perhaps fancy, Reform, but cholera. There is a great panic, as great a panic as I can remember, particularly in the City.'[3]

The bubble was, however, pricked at the end of June by a letter in *The Times* from Dr James Johnson, editor of the *Medico-Chirurgical Review*.

> It will hardly be doubted that the terrible malady cholera-phobia rages at this moment, epidemically, through every spot of the British Isles, and I am sorry to say that *The Times* journal has tended to spread and diffuse the contagion beyond that of every other vehicle. The choleraphobia will frighten to death a far greater number of Britons than the monster itself will ever destroy by his actual pestilence.[4]

Coming from an experienced and respected epidemiologist this letter effectively reduced the panic. Once the newspapers and journals refused to print material capable of generating alarm or giving credence to 'idle or knavish therapeutic speculations',[5] fear subsided. Greville wrote on 8 July that 'People are beginning to recover from their terror of the cholera, seeing that it does not come.'[6]

Choleraphobia was, therefore, transitory. In June 1831 it was the response of the propertied classes in London, possibly confined primarily to those who attended the London salons, to an external threat. It was an extreme reaction, most people continuing to act normally although keeping an eye open for possible danger, and reflected not only the threat from cholera but also fears for the general stability of society.[7]

The crucial catalyst for choleraphobia was the absence of reliable information concerning cholera's progress. Accurate and trustworthy news was at a premium in 1831 and the void was filled by rumours. Defined as 'a specific (or topical) proposition for belief, passed along from person to person, usually by word of mouth, without secure standards of evidence being present',[8] rumours exist in every society, however advanced. They are particularly common at times of uncertainty, when a major issue cannot be resolved with the information available. They flourish in a highly ambiguous situation, as during the period of the Great Fear in France in 1789.[9] Choleraphobia should be seen in this context, as rumours passed along the chains of communication. It came in waves, responding to every significant advance made by the disease. It reappeared with the publication of the 20 October Orders in Council and spread like wildfire when cholera was reported in Sunderland. Within a matter of days places as far from the North-East as Caernarvon, Gloucester, Norwich and Plymouth were suffering from choleraphobia. Similar reactions were observed when the horrific outbreak in Gateshead was reported at the end of December.[10] Indeed, the phenomenon seemed to increase in proportion to its distance from the seat of the disease. One correspondent to *The Times* noted that 'the Sunderland cholera made more noise at Newcastle than it does there, and perhaps more in London than at Newcastle'.[11]

Most newspapers obtained a national coverage of events at this period by the verbatim copying of news items from their rivals. When, as in the North-East, the local press deliberately played down the virulence of the disease, some editors were tempted to embellish what little information was available. One, for example, writing in December 1831 from a city more than four hundred miles from the infected region, felt free to state that 'if the sphere of the disease is now really so much extended [it was still confined to an area around Newcastle and Sunderland], there can be little hope of any part of the kingdom being long exempt from this formidable scourge of the human race'.[12] But even this paled into insignificance before the *Morning Chronicle*'s prophecy (made only a matter of days after cholera officially arrived in London and while *The Times* was denying its existence) that 'Before the cholera becomes extinct, death may close the mortal existence of one or two hundred thousand British Islanders, and twice that number may be subjected to the disease and the misery of protracted recovery.'[13] Even the well-intentioned, panic-reducing articles in newspapers were counter-productive, for, combined with the scaremongers', they merely intensified ambiguity.

Choleraphobia was, however, relatively harmless, although there were reports of people killing themselves by an excessive dependence on their favourite panacea. The phenomenon reflected genuine but general and diffuse alarm amongst the propertied classes. It was, according to one Sheffield newspaper, symptomatic of the English character. 'The truth is, that Englishmen of all other people on the face of the earth, tremble most at the approach of an enemy, and perhaps fear him least, when he is in actual combat.'[14]

It is important to distinguish these waves of fear from the reactions which occurred when cholera actually reached a community. Alarm was generated as the disease crept closer. The unprecedented outbreak in Gateshead 'involved the population of Newcastle and its suburbs in despair',[15] although Newcastle was already infected. When cholera reached Kirkintilloch, the inhabitants of neighbouring Glasgow became panic-stricken. 'You can form no idea of the alarm that is here at present; business and work are quite neglected.'[16] The greatest alarm was reserved for the moment cholera struck. This fear was not like choleraphobia, which spread pulsatingly from a particular source, but was local and a consequence of unambiguous, if embellished, information. It was to occur frequently in 1832, scattered both in time and place depending on cholera's diffusion. Nor was it confined only to the propertied classes, as choleraphobia seems to have been. In Newcastle the first case (that of Robert Jordan) precipitated general alarm, while at the Carron Iron Works in Falkirk in March 1832, everyone became frantic. 'I saw one poor girl last night literally frightened out of her life though in reality there was not much the matter with her . . .'[17] The unfortunate people of Hull had to undergo several false alarms and bouts of fear before the first official case occurred.[18] The greatest panic, however, was displayed in Gateshead.

> The inhabitants of Gateshead fell asleep on 25 December, in perfect security and devoid of panic, but before the sun rose on the 26th, fifty-five individuals had been seized, thirty-two of whom were destined not to see it set. For several days subsequent to the 27th, the panic of the inhabitants was greater than I have ever witnessed under any pestilence, while the new cases decreased . . .[19]

How people reacted to this fear depended on the options open to them.[20] Flight had been the eternal prerogative of the prosperous in times of pestilence. It was they who had the means and the ability to seek safety in their country seats or at watering places far from the main concentrations of the poor. Such a response was in evidence from the beginning of the epidemic. Many of the propertied in the North-East beat a hasty and somewhat undignified retreat in October and November 1831. The one major exception was Lord Londonderry who, with his wife and children, deliberately stayed in the region as an example to his more fainthearted brethren, many of whom had fled to London. Londonderry made appearances in Sunderland and Seaham several times a week whilst cholera was present. 'I felt that, had I abdicated and given way to alarm, the mischief that it would have occasioned in this country would have been incalculable. It would have been the tocsin for a general emigration.'[21] He accepted the perhaps old-fashioned view that responsibilities and duty to the community were an integral part of aristocratic privilege, which he was defending particularly strenuously in the House of Lords at this time.

The wealthy of London were expected to follow the example not of Londonderry but of his colleagues. The Duchess de Dino had written to Barante in March 1832, 'à la première personne de la société qui sera aux prises des hauts degrés du mal, je prévois que le sauve-qui-peut deviendra général'.[22] But London society did not flee in February 1832. The *Examiner* noted that there was no panic in London and Greville was relieved to discover that 'the cholera has produced more alertness than alarm here.'[23] The slow progress of the disease in the metropolis and its preference for the poor probably explained this reaction, but circumstances changed when cholera returned in July. Even amongst the first cases there was a significant number 'in easy and affluent circumstances' and yet the fatality rate remained as high as in the first outbreak.[24] The hint was taken and many people fled into the countryside, beginning the season of house parties earlier than usual.

> The appearance of the disease, so much increased in virulence, has tended to thin the west end of the town to a great extent of persons of property and distinction, and the thin attendance of both Lords and Commoners in Parliament affords proof of the desire of those who can do so, to leave town. . . . In fact, should Parliament not soon be prorogued, the business in the Commons will be at a standstill from the non-attendance of sufficient members to constitute a House.[25]

Greville perceptively put his finger on the reason for this. Having noted disapprovingly Daniel O'Connell's movement between Dublin and London as the disease 'appeared first at one and then the other place', he went on to write,

> Some servants of people well known have died, and that frightens all other servants out of their wits, and they frighten their masters; the death of any one person they are acquainted with terrifies people much more than that of twenty of whom they know nothing . . . when they hear that Lady such a one's nurse or Sir somebody's footman is dead, they fancy they see the disease actually at their own door.[26]

A fortnight later Greville was proved right. The death of the 'young and beautiful' Mrs Smith, 'dressed to go to church on Sunday morning . . . created a terrible alarm; many people have taken flight, and others are suspended between their hopes of safety in country air and their dread of being removed from metropolitan aid'.

This pattern can be seen elsewhere. It probably explains why some local board of health minutes peter out when the disease is present. Certainly it appears that the propertied fled when cholera was deemed a *direct* threat. This sometimes occurred after the disease had been present for several weeks in a community, for many local newspapers failed to report local outbreaks. In Plymouth, for example, the local newspaper did not mention the disease for a month and it was only when cholera was at its height that people began to flee.[27] In Bilston, 'those inhabitants who possessed the means' quit the town at a time when 'the pestilence was literally sweeping everything before it, neither age, nor sex, nor station escaping . . .' .[28] In Dumfries, where cholera began on 10 September, the mass exodus was on its way during the worst part of the epidemic, after 25 September. Complaints that the wealthy were fleeing York only became heard in the very week in which cholera reached its peak. Rumours of this became so exaggerated in London that the *Globe* reported the flight of 6,000 families from York, out of a total population of 26,000.[29] While evidence from other towns is not so specific, it does demonstrate that flight was a common response by many of the propertied classes.[30]

Nevertheless, the effects of such reactions perhaps should not be exaggerated. Because they occurred primarily when the disease was at its height in particular localities, their overall impact was relatively slight. The situation, for example, was not comparable with that of either Paris or Moscow, where flight was a much more widespread phenomenon. It was commonsense, rather than outright panic, which sometimes persuaded the wealthy to retreat to their country estates or to the spa towns. They could not, however, be assured of safety there. Bath, with its filthy dens and notorious mobs, did not escape the disease,[31] nor did the watering place of Askern. When, in August, a waiter died of cholera in Askern, the consequence was 'that this agreeable watering place, which was filling very fast, [was], as far as visitors and strangers [were] concerned, all but depopulated'.[32]

Flight was only one extreme response possible; another was to deny the existence of the disease. This was a common phenomenon, most particularly in the early stages of the disease in a community. Its most notorious occurrence was in the North-East in the late autumn of 1831. The attempted cover-up by the local ruling classes and the suborning of the local medical profession only came to light because of the fortuitous presence in Sunderland of the military surgeon James Butler Kell, who not only had witnessed cholera in Mauritius in 1829 but also personally knew Sir James McGrigor, then on Halford's Board of Health. Kell was very conscientious and soon became suspicious when four isolated cases of a disease similar to cholera occurred in August.[33] No official reports were made of these; it was only when Kell attended a meeting of the local board of health (of which he was an honorary member) on 30 August that he learned of the death of one Robert Henry, a pilot.[34] Inquiries having satisfied him that Henry had piloted a ship from the Baltic into harbour shortly before his death, Kell immediately, and without informing the Sunderland authorities, reported his fears to McGrigor in London.[35]

Kell's independent action and his subsequent complaints about the quarantine establishment angered the local authorities, but, primarily because of the few and isolated cases at this juncture, they were able to refute the surgeon's claims and silence the London Board of Health's inquiries with relative ease.[36] Five weeks elapsed before Kell heard of further cases, the first of which occurred close to where several ships were completing quarantine. Soon afterwards he learned, again by chance, of William Sproat Snr's death, which was subsequently to be accepted as the first cholera fatality in the British Isles. Kell once again informed London, although he later claimed to have asked a local clergyman to persuade George Robinson, chairman of the local board of health, to write to London. (No message was received from Robinson however.)[37]

Dr Reid Clanny, chairman of the medical subcommittee of the board of health, was also convinced of cholera's presence but he failed to obtain the agreement of his medical colleagues on the board. On 1 November, however, after several more fatal cases had been reported, a general meeting of the medical fraternity reversed this decision, with no dissenting voice. The local board reported this decision officially to London.[38]

When only one further case was reported in the next few days (the spasmodic incidence of cholera at the beginning of an epidemic is a common phenomenon), doubts were expressed as to the wisdom of the 1 November decision, especially as the implementation of quarantine regulations was certain to have unpopular economic repercussions. Of the thirty-five medical men practising in Sunderland, twenty-eight lived in the middle-class parish of Bishopwearmouth and were dependent on the good offices of their middle-class patients. They began to rue their hasty decision of 1 November.

Consequently, when the three government agents, Robert Daun, Lieutenant Colonel Michael Creagh and Doctor Gibson, arrived in Sunderland, they faced a growing conspiracy of silence, and Daun was soon at his wit's end. He could only confirm the presence of Asiatic cholera if he was given access to the victims, but professional etiquette prevented him from visiting the sick without permission from the attending doctor. Several times Daun waited in vain for a doctor to arrive. At first he charitably excused their non-appearance on the grounds of overwork, but he quickly realised the real reason for this obstructionism. 'It had been signified to [me] that the mercantile and shipping interest of this port, dreading that restriction might be imposed upon the commerce, are strongly opposed to the belief that cholera exists here in any unusual degree or form and that they are supported in this view of the case by not a few of the medical practitioners here.'[39]

Daun's views were confirmed by the moves of the commercial class to deny the existence of cholera. Letters to newspapers and 'official' circulars were part of this programme to discredit the local board of health. One handbill claimed that

> Any person supplying the Board of Health with a few cases of Asiatic cholera, will receive a liberal and substantial reward and should none such be obtainable any number of cases of British origin, however small, will be thankfully received and most gratefully acknowledged.
>
> The object of the advertisers being altogether public, unalloyed by any private or personal feelings, morbid desire of present profit, or selfish longings after future fame or advantage, they trust their fellow townsmen, placing all confidence in their disinterestedness and wisdom, will endeavour by every means in their power to get up a few appearances to save the credit of the Firm from the sneers of the credulous and the aspersions of the ignorant and malicious.

> Apply at the Commission Room at any hour, no questions will be asked and no mistake dreamt of.[40]

The commercial viewpoint was also spread privately to London. The merchant John Stevenson wrote to a relative on 9 November, 'The truth is that a set of alarmists of the surgeon order have made the most of a story which had of itself a dangerous aspect, and so industriously have some of them followed their advocations that cases of cholera have been made out of toothache, stabbing in the abdomen with a fork, jaundice, dropsy and every complaint in the vocabulary of disease . . .'.[41]

The real onslaught by the commercial classes came in the second week of November, when at a series of meetings a resolution condemning the erroneous reports sent to London and a motion in favour of publicly naming those doctors at the 1 November meeting were passed. This direct threat of intimidation was immediately successful. Of the nineteen medical practitioners who met that day to express their opinions on cholera, only one was prepared to defy the commercial interests by claiming the existence of Asiatic cholera. At least four of these doctors had previously attended cholera cases, and one had even suffered from the disease.[42] The rout was completed the next day when twenty-eight medical men signed a statement which, while admitting the presence of a disease with every symptom of epidemic cholera, stated that it was not contagious, had not been imported and would only be worsened by the pernicious effects of quarantine regulations.[43] Even Clanny signed the document, thus isolating Kell, although he had the excuse of having had his life threatened. Daun had informed the Central Board on the previous day that a mob of sailors was going to attack Clanny's house that evening.[44]

At the same time as the medical profession was wilting before the economic facts of life, the commercial and shipping interests turned their attention to the local board of health. At yet another meeting on the 11th, resolutions hostile to Kell, Clanny and George Robinson were passed and the local board was replaced by one more amenable to the pressure of specific interest groups. Daun informed London on the 15th that 'a new board of health has been constituted consisting of God knows how many members —a great proportion of them shipowners and merchants—on the ground forsooth that their interests must be represented on the board ! ! !'. This victory was made easier by the sudden death of George Robinson from English cholera.[45]

Several points are worth making on these proceedings. First, a specific interest group within the local ruling class found it comparatively easy to steamroller the dependent medical profession into submission. This is understandable, not only because of the threat to the profession's practices, but also because the major medical opponent to the commercial interests came from outside the charmed circle of the local power structure. Admittedly, when the local board of health had been first established in June, Kell had been well received and his opinions eagerly sought, but once he had given his primary allegiance to the Central Board and had failed to appreciate the strength of ideas on local autonomy and self-sufficiency, he was dropped. Thereafter he was fighting a losing battle, especially once Clanny, who also saw matters from a wider viewpoint, had been threatened.

Second, the commercial interests had to defeat another section of the ruling class before taking control of the local boards of health. Those who were to be overwhelmed in November represented in one sense, a more comprehensive range of interests than their narrowly-based opponents. They were a cross-section of all groups which made up the ruling elite : clergy, professional men, magistrates as well as the thrusting commercial groups, who saw their responsibilities in the wider context of the town as a whole. But in another sense the commercial interests represented a wider range of social groupings, in that the mass of the working classes equally needed free and unfettered trade for their livelihoods. Most of the able-bodied in Sunderland worked either as mariners, keelmen ('amphibious race, half landmen, half boatmen') or casters, occupations which at the best of times were dependent on the vagaries of the weather.[46] Any slowing down in trade as a result of quarantine would affect them, probably more than the commercial interests.

The third point worthy of note is that while the commercial interests could display naked power at the local level, they were ineffective when it came to dealing with the central authority. The Central Board, aware of the inefficiency of the Sunderland quarantine establishment (each ship had to pass through Sunderland to the quarantine station at Deptford), ensured that the new Sunderland board of health's pressure to abolish the regulations was ineffectual. The period of quarantine was cut from fifteen to ten days but this was due to the new information which Russell and Barry had sent back from Russia. Dire warnings of the results of widespread unemployment were equally unavailing. Hedworth Williamson of Whitturn Hall near Sunderland told Melbourne that unemployment would be high not just in Sunderland but also in the mining communities, if the coastal coal trade with London was interrupted. The colliers had, said Williamson, 'been for some time in an unsettled state and I cannot answer whether now they be well or ill affected towards their employers. . . . Should distress drive the numerous classes . . . to serious dissaffection and insubordination, is the military force now in this part of the country sufficient to preserve the peace and defend property?'[47] The central authority preferred, however, the evidence from their own representatives on the spot; not even Lord Londonderry could obtain relief for Seaham harbour.[48]

The reports which Daun, Creagh and eventually Barry sent from the North-East showed that while in theory the commercial interests had similar objectives to their workforce, the relief of the sick and needy was not high on the list of the new board's priorities. Without the exertions of a local clergyman, there would have been no cholera hospital in Sunderland. The new board laid more store by words than actions, doing their best to hinder the work of the government representatives. Even as late as January 1832, under the orders of the local board, more than one doctor was still refusing to give Daun daily reports on cholera cases.[49] Nor was anything done to relieve the manifest hardship from which many of the poor suffered. The bulk of the poor lived in the parish of Sunderland, from which even labourers, as soon as they felt economically secure, escaped. Thus the poor rate fell on only a small proportion of the population, who themselves were no more than small traders and 'incipient speculators'. The wealthy, by contrast, lived in the comparatively healthy parish of Bishopwearmouth, where the rate was low. Little was done to help the beleaguered poor, close to the river. David Barry suggested the issuing of a joint rate: 'The rich would thus be obliged to preserve from starvation and premature decay, the very instruments by which their fortunes were built up, but which in this place they desert when their fortunes reach a certain bulk.'[50] Such was the antipathy he knew this would cause that he sent his letter privately, 'lest it might come out with my name, before I can escape from here. The black diamond merchants would condemn me to the mines for such a suggestion. The blunt matter of fact however is, that they want to throw the poor upon government and save themselves from a legal rate being impressed upon them.'[51]

Denial of cholera in Sunderland brought to light not only the seamier side of working class living conditions, but also the rapacious and parsimonious face of capitalism. Any opposition to the dominant commercial interest was ruthlessly bludgeoned into submission. One visiting Londoner wrote to a colleague in January 1832, 'The people there [Sunderland] seem callous and indifferent to cholera; indeed some of our customers are infatuated enough to insist on it [being called] the Foreign Cholera, as if it had never been here.'[52] It is hard not to believe that late in 1831 it would have been foolhardy of any inhabitant of Sunderland to have adopted an alternative posture.

In Newcastle, the next major commercial centre to be infected, the same syndrome was repeated. On this occasion the mayor on his own initiative reported the first fatal case to London, an action with which the local board of health violently disagreed. Newcastle was placed under an immediate ten-day quarantine, which even a unanimous resolution from the medical profession denying cholera's existence failed to rescind. Sufficient pressure was put on the mayor for him to recant, but within four days further cases occurred which put the issue beyond doubt.[53]

The denial of cholera, while not confined to one socio-economic stratum,[54] was to be the major tool for those whose profits were threatened by goverment regulation in 1831–2. In Manchester, in December, the board of health, no doubt mindful of the experiences in the North-East, ordered that no medical man make public any case of cholera until the medical board had given their opinion.[55] In London, where the shipowners had called meetings of protest when the quarantine laws were invoked in June 1831, petty shopkeepers and artisans used their influence on local vestries to protect their personal interests. A reluctance to sanction a new rate and the fear that potential customers might be scared away were two factors influencing the shopkeeper/artisan viewpoint. In Christchurch, Surrey, for example, a majority of the vestry opposed any action by the local board of health in February 1832 and refused to sanction funds. Twice vestry meetings were adjourned *sine die* when this issue was raised, once after the Central Board had insisted on the vestry convening.[56] There is no evidence to confirm the establishing of a local board in St Clement Danes, although it is possible that their 'permanent committee of relief' may have temporarily functioned in this manner.[57] Certainly, the Central Board never received any information from this parish. In St Paul Covent Garden, an attempt to form a board of health when cholera had reached the metropolis was thwarted by radical petty tradesmen who passed an amendment which quoted verbatim the contents of a radical fly-poster which had been plastered throughout Lambeth a week previously and then reprinted in radical newspapers.[58] Advertising space in three newspapers was bought to broadcast the vestry's denial of cholera's presence so that 'an extinguisher may be put on the alarming and unjustifiable panic upon the subject of cholera so ruinous to trade and mercantile affairs'.[59]

Eventually the Central Board of Health ordered the formation of a board of health in the parish, but an attempt to give it powers and money was overwhelmingly defeated. An amendment, asserting the healthiness of the parish and pointing out that elsewhere cholera cases were merely amongst 'the half-starved poor' and that they were the responsibility of the Committee of Management, was passed by sixty-two votes to ten.

After a meeting with the Central Board, at which Pym expressed satisfaction with the parish's activities, the Committee of Management became the local board of health. An election for the committee took place, in which the three leaders of the anti-cholera party topped the poll. Those elected were from the small shopkeeper/artisan class. Two were potato salesmen; the others a locksmith, a baker, a laceman, a whipmaker, a woollen draper and a bootmaker.

The denial of cholera was possible, however, only in certain circumstances. It certainly helped to forestall panic amongst the commercial interests during cholera's first visit to London. The Duchess de Dino admitted in March, for example, that the commercial classes had remained calm. 'Ici, l'intérêt puissant du commerce a étouffé la terreur, et cette puissance est si réelle que personne à Londres n'a eu le courage d'avoir peur.'[60] But once several members of the Stock Exchange fell sick with cholera, the exodus began. Similarly in Bilston, prominent among those fleeing were the manufacturers, many of whose factories were closed down.[61] Eventually, therefore, personal safety came to mean more than the profit motive. Possible while cholera kept closely to one socio-economic class, the practice of denying it became untenable once the disease advanced up the social scale.

Flight and the denial of cholera were only the most extreme options open to the propertied in 1831–2. Most, possibly a majority of the middle ranks of society, did not respond in either way but came to terms with cholera by reference to their own social mores and religious mentalities. Sensible precautions could be taken without outright flight. The Marquis of Stafford, for example, fearful that his servants might be the means by which cholera invaded his London household, forbade them from going further east than Charing Cross. Tradesmen were refused entry to his grounds, while the postman threw his letters into the drive and his newspapers arrived from over the garden wall.[62] In Paisley, the unfortunate doctors were asked not to frequent the coffee room whilst treating cholera patients. And in a Glasgow reading room, gentlemen read through pocket spy-glasses, at a safe distance from possible infection. Others were seen stealing through the mud in the middle of the road, muffled up to the eyes, afraid of every breath they inhaled.[63] Social intercourse, though muted, therefore continued, except when the disease was at its height. Then, theatres closed down, assizes were postponed and some annual wakes cancelled.[64] The most graphic illustration of the dislocation at cholera's height came from Edward Allison in Dumfries, one of the worst hit towns in Scotland. Most of the shops were shut, the streets were covered with quicklime and

> the hearse was slowly traversing the various lanes and followed by the nearest friends of the deceased. . . . The panic was so great that several thousands of persons fled and during torrents, scarcely an individual was to be met in the streets—the medical men, gigs and the hearses only were to be seen or

> heard. It was truly melancholy and solemn to witness the deserted state of the town.[65]

Those who had not fled and were locked in the sanctuary of their homes probably spent much of their time trying to rationalise this catastrophic series of events. For many, the certitude of religious belief offered some comfort. Cholera could be seen as the vehicle of a vengeful God displaying His anger. What He was angry about depended on the individual conscience. Robert Southey, like his friend Robert Ferguson, saw cholera as a somewhat oblique warning against political reform and a sign that social parameters were dissolving. To an extent he was the victim of his own propaganda, for in 1829 he had, through the ghost of St Thomas More, warned that epidemics which had devastated London in previous centuries were still capable of returning. The breakdown of the old paternalistic social order had left an uncontrollable multitude of the wicked and the ignorant ready to pour out from the lanes and alleyways of the metropolis at the slightest provocation. By 1832, probably startled by the accuracy of the first part of his prediction, Southey had joined the Keswick board of health, but still feared that the poor would break loose.[66]

For others, cholera's presence justified their view that society was morally corrupt, the disease being the awful consequence of depraved habits such as drinking and smoking. The Leeds milliner Robert Ayrey wrote to his brother,

> I am sorry to say religion in Leeds has become in a state of lukewarmness this last three years but this plague or what is termed the cholera morbus perhaps is sent to stir the people up. . . . It appears to me that the Lord is scourging us as a nation for our multiplied sins . . . it ravages more especially the drunkards and the sabbath breakers.[67]

The evidence from nearly every local epidemic reinforced this claim, for the first victims were invariably the dissolute and the depraved. Hence the widespread increase in churchgoing throughout the country during the first months of the disease, so that an avenging God could clearly distinguish between the moral and the immoral. One York newspaper accurately forecast when the disease first broke out that it would have a good effect on 'the moral and religious deportment of all ranks of society'.[68] As a result there was 'a firmer tone to the consistent Christian . . . the scoffer has been silenced and the waverer confirmed; and our places of worship have been attended with much more numerous congregations'.[69] Religious observance in York had been in steep decline before 1832 (the rector of St Saviour's had estimated that two-thirds of the inhabitants never went to church at all), yet when on a Friday night in mid-July a divine service was held at St John's Micklegate, the congregation was 'so numerous that they could scarcely find standing room'.[70]

Similarly in rural Plympton, when the disease was gaining ground in August, a much larger congregation than usual assembled and twice the usual number received the sacraments. 'A marked solemnity of deportment prevailed.' Yet within a week, as cholera burgeoned, the numbers declined dramatically, 'owing to the absence of some of the principal families, the sickness of many, or the fear of assembling which prevailed among others'.[71]

The epidemic seems not to have led to millenarian movements, although Thomas Arnold, deeply depressed by the rural disturbances of 1830 and the Reform Bill crisis, began to see signs of the end of the world when cholera broke out.[72] Religious revivals there were, however. One, begun in September 1831 by John Elias in north Wales, was helped by the cholera. In Denbigh in July 1832 the big chapel known as Capel Canol was filled with serious looking worshippers at seven in the morning. On the following Sunday, over 700 attended the local Methodist Sunday School. Similarly in Merthyr in late September the local Wesleyan minister William Rowlands held several prayer meetings in conjunction with other denominations which were very well attended.[73] The Primitive Methodists also made rapid strides during the epidemic. Great revivals accompanied the cholera in Sunderland and South Shields, while the Kendal circuit reported an increase of 600 members, a phenomenal number by the standards of the time.[74]

In an age when religious forms and observances were still of importance, religion played a major part in reducing panic. It offered comfort and security in a rapidly changing and dangerous world and enabled a totally illogical and mystifying phenomenon to be explained. 'It is in the ineffable potency of the Great

Jehovah to hurl down at his might behest his weapons of destruction, totally imperceptible to our senses.'[75] It also, perhaps paradoxically, supplied a base from which the disease could be counterattacked. Both clergy and laity, although frequently adopting a high moral tone when considering cholera victims, fought the disease with the only means at their disposal, with charity, commonsense and no little faith. The exertions of the Reverend William Leigh of Bilston and Charles Girdlestone of Sedgeley as their congregations were decimated in the holocaust are only the best known examples of the Christian ethic in practice. William Coppard in Plympton, Vaughan Thomas in Oxford and John Robinson in York, as well as a host of clergymen of all denominations who worked on the local boards, visited the sick and buried the dead, demonstrating a sense of pastoral duty which can be compared favourably with that of the next generation of incumbents such as Dean Hook and Edward Jackson of Leeds.[76] Even Henry Philpotts, the much maligned anti-Reform Bishop of Exeter, did not shirk his duty as the radicals claimed. He returned to Exeter when the disease broke out there and performed a confirmation ceremony in Plympton while the cholera was raging (as the service ended Coppard left to attend three new cases).[77]

We should not, perhaps, overstate the piety or exaggerate the beneficial effects of religion; the combating of cholera amongst the poor might be seen more as a means of defending the social order than as pure altruism. It is plausible that those who professed evangelical principles, as well as giving proof of their regeneration by good works, used cholera as an excuse to move amongst the poor, distributing useful and moral literature, although such actions certainly required courage and religious conviction. Nor were acts of charity, administered by, for example, the Bristol Anti-Cholera Association,[78] more than merely palliative. Nevertheless, it is worth emphasising that charity, whether from philanthropic bodies or from local boards of health, was better than nothing. The choice of beneficiary may have been determined by recourse to the middle-class distinction between the deserving and the undeserving poor, but without charity, as the Reverend Leigh said, 'Famine must have completed what pestilence had begun.'[79]

The foregoing analysis may be summed up as follows. It seems likely that, with regard to their perceptions of cholera, the propertied classes can be divided into several groups, determined by their general interest in foreign affairs, their economic function, and their relationship to power at the local level. By interest in foreign affairs is meant a relative awareness of events on a global scale and access to reasonably accurate sources of evidence. The first outburst of choleraphobia in June 1831 reflected the broad general awareness, by London society, of international events. This is not to suggest that they were necessarily more knowledgeable of European happenings than other social groups (the widespread interest in the events of the French Revolution in 1830 and in Belgium in 1832 belies that); rather, being in close contact with central government circles, they were privy to somewhat more, if still ambiguous, information on the possible consequences of cholera's progress through Europe. Choleraphobia's recrudescence in October and November 1831 was a consequence of the disease's arrival in an 'awareness zone' applicable to a larger proportion of the propertied classes; it had moved from the international to the national zone.

The general fear and dismay of choleraphobia gave way to sharper reactions when the disease entered the local zone of people's perceptions. It is at this level that economic and political considerations become relevant, for responses could be divergent, some people denying the existence of the disease, some fleeing from it, some doing both, and some ostensibly not reacting at all. Those who denied it did so because of personal economic considerations; their influence on events at the local level being determined by their relationship to the local power structure. Shipowners and artisans in some of the London parishes, had one thing in common; their hands on the levers of local power. Denial became, as it were, official ideology in those areas where economic interests, dependent on markets subject to dislocation by either anti-cholera measures or cholera's actual presence, controlled the local power structure. The apparent absence of the denial syndrome in other London parishes, for example, did not reflect different perceptions amongst the shopkeeper/artisan strata there; rather, in many parishes they did not control local resources and were not dominant in the local ruling class. Once cholera evidently reached a locality, however, and especially once deaths occurred amongst various socio-economic groups, the denial syndrome became redundant and economic interests were superseded by concern for private safety.

The concept of a local awareness zone also helps to explain the timing of the propertied classes' flight away from the disease. As mentioned above, flight occurred when cholera was felt to be a direct threat to life, usually occurring at the height of each local epidemic when fatalities began to occur amongst the wealthy and respectable. In contrast to the poor, who responded most emphatically when the disease *first* broke out in a community, the propertied seemed actually to become less alarmed at this point. It is obviously extremely difficult to plot fluctuations in fear, and any conclusions must remain tentative, but a letter from a Sunderland resident, written after the disease had been in the town for several months, possibly charts accurately changes in mood amongst the propertied. 'At the first', he wrote, 'many people were afraid of a contagious tendency; the experience of a week greatly removed their apprehension, but after further acquaintance, a more general belief prevails that, under certain circumstances, which are partly inexplicable, [cholera] is communicable.'[80]

This suggests a pattern of moods which seems to have been reflected in action: choleraphobia as a premature response to the prospect of a contagious disease; relative calm when the disease first arrives (either because of relief that the disease is confined to the poor or because of ignorance caused by the newspapers' failure to report the epidemic); and a determination to withdraw to safety (either by flight or by remaining within doors) when cholera's move up the social scale strongly suggests the presence of a communicable disease.

It is clear, therefore, that the responses of the propertied to cholera in 1832 fluctuated according to many circumstances, and that any analysis which presupposes a uniformity and simplicity of response underestimates the complexities involved in reaching an understanding of mentalities in the past.

7

The People and the Cholera: (i) The People, Authority and the Medical Profession

TERROR, panic, fear, alarm, fright and dread were all words used to describe people's reactions to the prospect and impact of cholera in 1832. Their value, as measurable and precise terms, especially in an historical context, is difficult to determine, for one man's terror is another man's alarm. Few, however, would argue with the proposition that the fear of death—and the fear of dying—are universal, innate phenomena. Not surprisingly, therefore, fear has always been the handmaiden of disease, throughout the ages. René Baehrel, for example, has written that, 'Toutes ces épidémies [from 1721 to 1884] provoquaient la Peur, une peur que les historiens ne mentionnent jamais qui certainement fut aussi grande que la Grande, une peur qui, pour reprendre le terme du fabuliste, était terreur . . .' .[1]

As mentioned in the previous chapter, the options open to the threatened or fearful were limited: one could fly from the threat or one could combat it. Flight could take several forms: either as a physical departure from the threatened environment; a withdrawal into one's home (essentially a passive response); or a denial of the threat's existence (the flight into unreality). Methods of combat also differed; one could join a local board of health; contribute to a charity; or nurse the sick. All these options were open to the ruling classes, whose wealth, status and prestige gave them a choice. This cannot be said for the poor, for physical flight or withdrawal from society could be achieved only at the expense of their livelihoods and what little security they possessed. Nor were they allowed the opportunity of emotional release which membership of a local board of health or a charity organisation gave to the ruling classes. In summary, they could deny cholera's existence and they could nurse the sick, neither of which could be expected to reduce tension. The former was unrealistic when there was evidence of people dying in the neighbourhood in a new and horrific way; the latter was disillusioning when adequate resources or knowledge were unavailable and was, moreover, possible only when the disease was present. It could not combat the fear of the *prospect* of cholera, during the stage of greatest uncertainty and tension.

Combat which relieved tension was, however, possible if the will o' the wisp cholera could be displaced, blamed on someone or something. The degree of unknowingness and ambiguity could be reduced by finding a scapegoat that could be used as a basis for explanation. In this way, not only were tensions reduced but the source of pre-existing tensions exposed, for the scapegoat is never chosen at random, but for reasons of logic. In France, argues Baehrel, popular reactions to the fear of cholera resulted in the development of a conspiracy theory, with the ruling classes, aided and abetted by the medical profession, plotting to kill off the surplus population. 'La haine contre le chirurgien, c'était la manifestation la plus nette de la haine de classe.'[2]

Louis Chevalier, seeking 'to obtain a knowledge of everything in people's behaviour which is intimately connected with the structure, needs, imperatives and functions of their body',[3] has argued that the cholera epidemic in Paris in 1832 brought forth the biological antagonisms which constantly simmered below the surface of Parisian society. Cholera emphasised biological facts and heightened the social tension resulting from internal contradictions within the Parisian social structure. Cholera was

> une catastrophe exceptionelle évidemment, mais résultant d'une situation normale—la condition des masses populaires—et révélant, d'autre part, en ces troubles eux-mêmes, le comportement habituel et la physionomie véritable de cette population. . . . Le choléra précise les fondements biologiques des antagonismes des classes . . .[4]

The disease, Chevalier feels, played a significant role in the political riots of April and June 1832 in Paris, although it did not *cause* them. Those of April grew from disturbances among rag and bone men, while the June uprising began when the funeral of General Lamarque degenerated into a republican insurrection. But the barricades went up in those very streets most affected by cholera. The disease, by heightening pre-existing social tension, helped to fuse what Hugo called 'la maladie politique et la maladie sociale'.

The emphasis which both Baehrel and Chevalier have put on cholera's ability to strip away the veneer of civilisation and lay bare the structural inequalities of society raises important issues for the study of cholera in Britain. In particular it opens for debate the question of a society's ability to absorb an epidemic situation, to survive the eruption of subterranean forces through the fissures created by the fracturing of social disciplines. The ideas and mentalities of the poor and dispossessed, those who bore the brunt of the disease and were the gravest threat to social order, are central to any analysis of this question. How they responded to cholera; what inequalities or disjunctions they perceived as the disease threatened to undermine their social norms; where they sought salvation; whom they blamed, are core problems for solution. The evidence available to explain motivation is diffuse, frequently impressionistic and sometimes refracted by the intercession of middle-class observers. By studying, however, the *actions* of the poor under stress, we can move closer to an understanding of how the trauma of cholera was accommodated into their *weltanschaung*. The crucial activities requiring analysis are the thirty riots and disturbances reported between February and November 1832 which related in some way to the presence of cholera (see Table 7.1). Varying considerably in intensity, from what contemporaries called 'petty tumults', in which small groups of people hurled stones and assaulted doctors, to large-scale riots involving hundreds, these incidents represented one way the poor could combat cholera. Their objective, distribution and intensity demonstrate where the dominant culture was pressing most strongly on the poor's sub-culture. Underlying it all, of course, lay the fear of the unknown and the fear of death, but in seeking to overcome atavistic fear, surrogates became the objects of attack.

One of the first fears to gain hold amongst the poor was that the disease was contagious. In accepting this proposition they were merely adhering to their traditional view of disease. Both the plague, although now no more than folk-memory, and smallpox were recognised as contagious.[5] It is unlikely that non-contagionist ideas had spread down the social scale at this stage, when they were still only a minority opinion among the

Table 7.1

Place	Date	Object of attack					Slogans						Damage				
		Doctors	Hospital	Attendants	Churchyard	Other	Burkers	Poisoning	Dissection	Denial	Gentlemen	Burial Rights	Slight	Serious	Police	Troops	Irish
Glasgow	Feb.		*				*	*					*				
Glasgow (Greenock)	March	*	*		*			*							*		
Glasgow (Gorbals)	March	*															
Edinburgh	March			*									*				
Edinburgh	May			*													
Greenwick	March			*													
Cathcart	April	*		*									*				
Paisley	Feb.	*				*		*	*								
Paisley	March	*	*	*					*					*	*	*	*
Dumfries	Nov.					*											*
London (Marylebone)	March	*		*			*								*		
[illegible]	July					*			*								

Liverpool (Toxteth Park)	June	*				*	*						*		*		
Liverpool (Oxford St Nth.)	June			*											*		*
Liverpool (Lime St)	June					*	*										
Liverpool (Vauxhall Rd)	June	*					*								*		
Liverpool (Vauxhall Rd)	June		*												*		*
Liverpool (Vauxhall Rd)	June			*											*		
Liverpool (Chisenhale St)	June			*											*		
Liverpool (Chisenhale St)	June			*								*			*		
Birmingham	August				*	*		*				*			*		
Bristol	August		*		*			*	*		*				*		
Leeds	June		*					*									
Sheffield	July			*					*			*					
Exeter (James St)	July				*							*					
Exeter (St. David's)	July				*												
Exeter (Rackclose Lane)	August.			*								*			*		
Manchester (Knott Mill)	July		*					*									
Manchester (Swan Street)	Sept.		*			*		*						*	*	*	*

medical profession. The poor's own experiences would have confirmed these contagionist beliefs, which the responses of the dominant culture further justified. The repeated visits of the district committees of the local boards of health, which in one way gave reassurance, in another raised suspicions. Concern for the poor had rarely been shown in this way before; did it mean that the middle-classes perceived some personal danger likely to arise from the poorer quarters?

The proliferation of posters and placards on walls all over town generated further alarm. Their message, although well-intentioned, was difficult to execute. Given the opportunity the poor would doubtless have been willing to keep their clothes and bed linen constantly cleaned and aired, but the basic requirements of a good water supply and fresh air were frequently unavailable. Whitewashing one's walls suggested that the cause of disease lurked in one's own dwelling. The posters were encouraging; all would be well if the recommendations were carried out. But the corollary, that failure to act would lead to unpleasant consequences, was more significant for the poor. Even the most blasé could not fail to realise that they were most at risk.

Moreover, the continual reference to looseness of the bowels as a warning sign could only have increased stress (and thereby possibly diarrhoea) in an age when bowel disorders were arguably the greatest single source of illness. This was noted in Lambeth in February 1832.

> The people of the house where the deaths occurred, and the neighbours, are in great tribulation in consequence of the ill-judged statements made about the cholera, and the placards specifying symptoms. Their fears are excited. Several complained that they felt ill and sick at heart. One poor woman who was suckling said her milk was disordered in consequence ...[6]

An inability to understand the posters' message also generated fear, for the language was frequently beyond the comprehension of the illiterate or semi-literate poor. Gaulter noticed in Manchester that the perpetual appearance of notices headed in bold and threatening letters CHOLERA increased alarm. At every corner the word *cholera* struck the eye; if one read further, contagion was obviously a factor requiring serious consideration.

Fear of cholera and of its contagious properties was therefore exacerbated by the actions and responses of the ruling classes. Flight, one response to this fear, was not available to the poor unless they were prepared to risk what small security and comfort they possessed. Equally, however, fear of contagion did not result in the extreme response of rioting, for not one of the reports of the riots mentions this as a precipitating factor. Faced with the possibility of a contagious disease the poor turned inwards, onto their own community. Unable to flee, they could at least isolate the sick and their relatives, who became pariahs. In Manchester the neighbours of one victim insisted that he be taken to hospital, against the wishes of his relatives.[7] In Gateshead in December (before the massive outbreak) a man could be seen tramping the streets looking 'miserably haggard'. His wife and two sons had died of cholera and, because these had been the first cases, his family was held responsible for the disease's presence. The persecution of his neighbours drove him away into the streets.[8] The scapegoating of bereaved relatives was relatively common. When one of the first fatal cases in Allen's Court, Manchester occurred (the court was soon to be devastated), the inhabitants 'could hardly be restrained from laying violent hands on [the victim's] widow.'[9] In Sedgeley the daughter of one of the first to die was left to fend for herself for two hours, screaming with pain and terror, before the local curate induced the neighbours to tend to her.[10] Again in Manchester, a man whose three children were in hospital was driven from his court by neighbours and then forced to flee from his brother's house, where he had sought sanctuary.[11] On occasion even relatives abandoned the sick, as in Musselburgh and Exeter, although such behaviour was exceptional in the Devon town.[12]

Under certain circumstances, therefore, and the evidence suggests these to be at the beginning of an epidemic when tension and uncertainty were high, fear of contagion could break down community feeling and even family ties. But the scapegoats were chosen from the community itself and not from the ruling classes. Lizars was correct in believing that

> The doctrine of contagion hardens the heart—destroys the finer and more amiable feelings of our nature; the kindly affection of the father for his family is blunted or destroyed;

> the still stronger link of nature between the mother and her offspring is broken, and she looks on her innocent children as sources of danger.[13]

The other reflex response of the middle-classes, to deny cholera's existence, was also open to distortion by the poor. To *hear* that cholera was being denied or that it was summer diarrhoea and not contagious, and yet to *see* all the preparations being taken (especially the establishment of temporary hospitals), heightened ambiguity. There may have been ulterior motives behind the desire to separate the sick poor from their friends and relatives. Certainly, central to ten of the disturbances under discussion was the question of removing victims to hospital and ten others involved incidents at hospitals. In Greenwick and Liverpool there is evidence to suggest that the poor refused to believe in cholera's existence. In the former town this opinion lasted only long enough to prevent one man from being removed from his home by medical attendants. Once deaths occurred in the home which could not be blamed on the doctors, feelings died down.[14] Regarding Liverpool the *True Sun* reported on 31 May,

> Nothing particular has occurred here, excepting that the lower orders are much enraged at the establishment of the cholera hospital, and have proceeded to some acts of outrage. In fact, people cannot be brought to believe that cholera exists in this town.[15]

Four incidents in Liverpool, occurring on 1 and 2 June and involving attacks on medical attendants and the hospital, may have been influenced by this belief. The first disturbance began when a sick man and his wife were being taken from their home in Perry Street to the hospital. A crowd of men and boys, estimated at a thousand strong, pursued the cholera cart to the hospital where, shouting 'Bring out the burkers, there go the murderers,' they hurled stones and forced the doctors to flee. Several passers-by were also assaulted. With the local police conspicuously absent, the disturbance was not quelled until a detachment of police from another part of Liverpool arrived to break it up.[16]

On the same day a crowd in Oxford Street North prevented

hospital porters removing a sick man whose wife had just died. The police arrived and dispersed the crowd, four people being arrested. These were: William Gunnall, 18; Peter McCann, 24; Ann Bradley, 33; and Jame M'Travis, 19. Gunnall was English, the rest Irish.[17] Also on 1 June a poor woman seen leaving the Lime Street cholera hospital yard was attacked by a crowd calling her 'a burker'. One can only presume that she had permitted a relative to be taken to hospital and that her 'friends' objected.

On the next day, 2 June, a surgeon walking down Vauxhall Road was informed of the presence of a sick woman in a nearby house. He recommended calling in the parish surgeon who discovered on his arrival that the body (the woman having presumably died in the meantime) had been hidden. A crowd then attacked the surgeon claiming that 'The doctors merely wanted to get the poor into their clutches to Burke them.' The police intervened to save the man from excessive harm. That evening a crowd assembled around the local cholera hospital was dispersed by the police, but only following an affray which led to several arrests. The crowd 'chiefly consisted of low Irish'.[18]

The paradoxical situation whereby a dominant ruling class response seemed to contradict its own actions may well have played a role in these early disturbances in Liverpool. As in Greenwick, however, it was an enigma which lasted only as long as victims were not dying in their own homes. How widespread these feelings were is uncertain, but they also existed in London and of course in the North-East.[19] It would appear that this response amongst the poor was a temporary phenomenon in merchant-intensive towns and cities where middle-class propaganda was most common. It was, however, transient and did not play a significant part in most of the disturbances in 1832.

Once cholera had settled in a community other actions by the ruling classes influenced the responses of the poor. For example, one of the local boards' regulations was that all materials capable of harbouring infection should be confiscated. Objections to this frequently resulted in petty tumults.[20] The 21 October Order in Council suggested that all old rags, clothes and hangings should be destroyed and that the victim's clothes and furniture 'should be submitted to copious effusions of water and boiled in a strong ley'. No mention was made of compensation for surviving relatives.[21] In practice the local boards took this part of the regulations very seriously and included the victims' clothes in the articles destroyed. This vigour compares unfavourably with the token lip-service sometimes paid to those regulations which entailed the expenditure of rates (nor is there evidence to suggest that the ageing Lord Amesbury's clothing was destroyed when he died of cholera). Compensation was, however, sometimes paid to the surviving family, not because it was their due but because otherwise offending articles were likely to disappear.[22] To be fair to the local boards, they might have thought that no one would have wanted to keep 'decayed articles', but for many of the poor, such as those Southwark Irish who were 'almost in a state of nudity, and are compelled to keep within doors; these are poor widows with their destitute children', they would have been a boon.[23]

A lack of respect for the property rights of the poor was one thing; a more important attack on their rights came with the regulations which required a swift burial after death from cholera. This was to strike deeply both at the poor's fundamentalist Christian doctrine and at their perceptions of what constituted a socially and culturally acceptable style of dying. The Order compelling burial within twelve hours was not issued until 13 July 1832, but long before then local magistrates, encouraged by the local boards and the Central Board of Health, had acted on this question.

Opposition to this regulation developed along two lines, one relating to the disruption of traditional death ceremonials and the other to the dread of premature interment. Burial within hours of death struck deeply at the traditional demands of the poor for a highly structured burial ritual. While it is difficult to assess exactly how important ritual was for the poor, the widespread desire for a 'good send-off' reflected in the popularity of friendly societies and burial clubs and the horror at the prospect of a pauper funeral both suggest that the solemnity and the ceremonials, if not the religious purposes, of the burial ritual were of fundamental importance, both psychologically and socially.[24] For the survivor, death causes ambivalent emotions, the desire to give way to fear and horror combining with the desire to pay homage to the dead. If the survivor gives way to fear and flees, material civilisation is threatened. Death 'threatens the very cohesion and solidarity of the group, and upon this depends the organisation of that society, its tradition, and finally the whole culture'.[25] Funeral rites have an important function to perform in counteracting the centrifugal forces of fear, dismay and demoralisation. They provide the most powerful means of reintegrating the group's shaken solidarity and the re-establishment of morale. Funeral rites ensure the victory of tradition and culture.[26]

It was, therefore, important that the traditional ritual over the dead should be pursued. In many places the poor were expected to touch the corpse as a token that they wished him no ill and were at peace and amity with him.[27] This, as well as a morbid curiosity, could explain why the poor continued to visit the houses of the dead in 1832, even against medical advice.[28]

The most widely observed part of the burial ritual was the 'lykewake' or wake. Wakes, it has been said, endorse and duplicate the feelings of the survivors, creating 'a social event out of a natural act'.[29] They, of course, extended the period between death and burial. In Kent it was customary not to bury the dead until seven or eight days had elapsed. In Wolverhampton, the poor preferred funerals on a Sunday, 'arising either from the holiness of the day or from convenience as not interfering with their laborious pursuits'.[30] It was, however, the Irish who used the wake as a key part of the funeral ritual, with symbolic games and plays, the consumption of much food and drink, together with prayer and mourning.[31] It was they who seemingly most objected to swift burial. During the epidemics in Liverpool and London the poor Irish frequently tried to keep the bodies of the dead from the authorities. One such disturbance in Liverpool, that of 2 June, has already been mentioned. On 10 June a riot occurred after a surgeon visited a patient in a cellar in Chisenhale Street. The patient was willing to go to hospital and his wife agreed, if assurance were given that the body would be returned for the wake (such was the apparent confidence in which the medical profession was held). The surgeon could not promise this, however. He eventually only escaped from the house with great difficulty and on the way to the hospital the empty cholera cart was attacked in Great Howard Street by a crowd of men and boys. The police arrived and 'a respectable looking man, dressed in black, was taken into custody, for overturning the palanquin, and conveyed to Bridewell'. He was bailed at £50 to appear at the next sessions.[32]

Threats and cajolery were sometimes used to prise the corpse from the grips of relatives. Bribes were occasionally effective, as in Tottenham where Rowland Hill, later to be famous for the penny post, told the obstinate relatives of one victim that 'if the corpse reach the churchyard by 2 o'clock they shall have a sovereign for the wake'. The body arrived on time and was immediately buried.[33]

Generally, the onus of persuading the Catholic poor to accept swift burial was put on the clergy. In March 1832 Greville asked the Reverend Dr Branston to draw up an address against waking, which the Privy Council offered to print and circulate.[34] It is doubtful if this had much effect, for in July the Catholic chapel in Finsbury Square was still receiving coffins from all over the City, which were not being interred until the Sunday. The mass grave was left open until filled, which drove one irate neighbour to write, 'I hope the day is not distant when the inhabitants of this wealthy City will not imitate a certain maniac of old, "who had his dwelling among the tombs . . .".'[35]

Traditional ritual processes continued beyond the period of waking and these too were disrupted by the demand for swift burial. When the disease reached its height the plans for the efficient and decorous burial of the dead frequently broke down and the horrors of the plague years were renewed with the digging of large pits into which bodies were hastily thrown. In Musselburgh the disease spread so rapidly that a special pit was prepared, the first customer being the gravedigger himself.[36] In Bilston between thirty and forty people were buried each day in a huge pit when the epidemic was at its height. Here, probably uncharacteristically, the degradation of death was no respecter of status. 'Some who would not condescend to sit together in the same seat in the house of worship are thrown promiscuously into a grave, without coffins or shrouds.'[37] In Sheffield the dead at first were thrown into large graves in St George's churchyard, but from August the dead were carried, four or five at a time, on an opensided cart to unconsecrated ground.[38] Many of these new graveyards were unconsecrated and although Charles Pearson, chairman of the City of London board of health, believed that 'a large body of professing Christians of various denominations do not require their last resting place on Earth to be consecrated with any particular rites',[39] in fact to be buried thus carried a stigma, for only particular malefactors such as suicides did not have this right. Moreover, it raised the question whether physical resurrection at the Last Judgement was possible when a body was buried in unconsecrated ground. Disturbances occurred around this issue. On 6 March a young man died in the Greenock cholera hospital. A rumour spread that he had been poisoned by the doctors. To reduce tension the authorities offered to carry out a postmortem, but while this was acceptable to the boy's father, the crowd were angry because he was not permitted to be present during the examination. When the presiding doctor left the building he was pelted with stones by women (the physician in question, Dr Kirk, had already annoyed the local womenfolk by saying in a public lecture that they were 'nasty in their habits').

Another rumour then spread through the crowd. The boy was not to be buried in the churchyard but at night on an unconsecrated hilltop outside town. A crowd assembled again at the hospital to enforce a Christian burial. Local magistrates and police forcibly removed the body and buried it in unconsecrated ground and after uttering threats against the hospital, the crowd dispersed.[40]

To be the first buried in a new graveyard, unconsecrated or not, was also regarded with horror. In Devon it was believed that the devil seized the first corpse so buried, and frequently new graveyards lay empty until a passing stranger or tramp died who could then be offered as the sacrificial victim. Certainly in Exeter in 1832 there was great difficulty obtaining the first body to bury in the new Bury Meadow graveyard. To persuade the relatives of the deceased that a body was already interred, the gravedigger had partially to reopen the first grave and cut off some of the cloth covering the coffin. Similar beliefs were prevalent elsewhere, as far afield as Scotland.[41]

Other normal parts of the burial ritual were curtailed at this time. During the height of the epidemic the tolling of the church bell was forbidden. Some, a minority, of clergymen failed to carry out their duties. In Exeter one clergyman celebrated the service 'over' a body from outside the graveyard, signalling with a plumbline when the time came for lowering the body into the grave. At the Woolwich hulks the Reverend Samuel Watson refused to bury the dead until six bodies had accumulated and he then read the service on deck—a mile from the burial patch on the marshes—dropping his handkerchief when the time came for the bodies to be lowered. The practice of carrying underhand was widely unpopular and was one of the causes of the disturbance in the Southernhay graveyard in Exeter, where the crowd shouted that the victims were being buried like dogs.[42]

Opposition to the regulations compelling swift burial also arose owing to the fear of premature interment. This fear was common in the eighteenth and nineteenth centuries and rumours of such events were frequent. Cholera epidemics were particularly prone to amplify these fears because of the need for swift burial,[43] and the 1832 epidemic was no exception. In 1832 *The Times* reported two cases of premature interment, one of a boy who kicked the coffin lid while being taken for burial, the other of a man who threatened to kill anyone who tried to nail down his wife's coffin lid. Both 'victims' were later reported to be alive.[44] Similarly, *The Examiner* retold a story from *The Globe* concerning the death from cholera of a woman and her son in Old Street, Islington. The son was buried, but the old woman regained consciousness as the coffin lid was being hammered down. The son's grave was immediately opened and the body was found upside down with the face 'torn in agony'.[45]

These examples, apocryphal or not, were the result, not the cause, of rumours spreading along the rumour chain. Fear and rumour were mutually reinforcing, fear engendering rumours which in turn extended fears. The first rumours began in Sunderland where it was believed that the doctors, fearful of the disease, were stupefying their patients with laudanum and sending them off for burial while still alive.[46] It was said of Gateshead that

> All the bodies are buried in less than twelve hours after dissolution, some in two or three hours. The common people firmly believe the doctors stupefy their patients with laudanum and then hurry them off to the grave while yet alive and that they have dissected living bodies; many well-informed people too, think some have been interred alive.[47]

These rumours were founded on some 'logic'. Both physiological symptoms and the effects of some drugs gave credence to these rumours. Acute muscular spasms were a common symptom of cholera and they frequently persisted after death.[48] This was graphically illustrated in Haddington when a victim was about to be buried.

> The man was immediately invested with the usual habiliments of death.... The first thing the man did, was by the sweep of his right arm, to throw the grave cloths from his breast. A few fir boards were hastily nailed together for his coffin.... From the period of his reputed demise until the clods of the valley covered him, a space of little more than five hours elapsed.[49]

Some plans of treatment favoured by medical men also had similar disconcerting results. Opium and laudanum in large quantities, for example, could induce coma and symptoms similar to death, such as imperceptible breathing, heartbeat and pulse, and dilated eyes. Inexperienced or frightened medical men may well have incorrectly diagnosed death in such circumstances. For this they were not blameworthy, for many of the sick frequently lay in a comatose state for hours before death, whether or not they had been treated with opiates. Moreover, the relative backwardness of forensic science ensured that even the most attentive doctors would have had difficulty pronouncing death, in the somatic as well as the cellular sense. Early nineteenth-century textbooks on forensic science defined death in a vague and ambiguous manner. J. G. Smith, for example, wrote in 1821,

> If we are aware of what indicates life, which everyone may be supposed to know, though perhaps no one can say that he truly and clearly understands what constitutes it, we at once arrive at the discrimination of death. It is the cessation of the phenomena with which we are so especially familiar—the phenomena of life.[50]

The irreversible process of putrefaction was the only sure way of proving death, a highly unsuitable method during the presence of a disease which many authorities thought to be highly infectious.

Burial within twelve hours of death caused great distress and led to widespread defiance. It led logically on to suspicions concerning the medical profession. Thus during the epidemic fears that the doctors were murdering their patients spread throughout the country. They began in Sunderland where, according to Greville, the commercial classes explained the increased number of deaths by reference to the medical profession's need for bodies on which to practise morbid anatomy. The rumours soon received horrific embellishments. Daun reported the widespread belief that patients were being dissected before death and that one woman was cut up whilst begging to be spared.[51] Whether or not the ruling classes were unscrupulous enough to play on the poor's fears, rumours did begin to circulate soon after the postmortem examination of one of the first victims. As a result, the sick did not seek medical aid until too late, only agreeing to enter hospital when little could be done for them. With the recovery rate in the hospitals thereby being lower than amongst those who remained at home, the rumours gained credence. In Newcastle, when between twenty and forty cases a day were being reported, only three or four were actually entering hospital.[52]

In nearly all the riots of 1832 the object of attack was to be the medical profession. Either the doctors themselves were assaulted, or the hospitals in which they worked were attacked, or attempts were made to prevent the sick from falling into the doctors' clutches. Suspicion and fear of the medical profession was general, occurring in Hull, Dewsbury, York, Plymouth, Falkirk, Swansea and Droitwich, as well as in the towns which suffered riots. In Hull it was believed that a woman had been murdered in the cholera hospital so that her body could be dissected. In Falkirk the doctors were called 'resurrectionist vagabonds'. In York, Dewsbury and Plymouth the doctors were deliberately killing patients in order to claim a reward from the authorities (cured patients presumably did not count towards total fees). In Droitwich, the doctors were poisoning their patients. One man swore he would 'run the spit through' any doctor who entered his house. His wife died unattended.[53]

The key to the cholera riots in 1832, therefore, lies in the ambivalent attitude of the poor to the medical profession. It was ambivalent because the doctors had a major role to play in the crisis as agents of relief and therapy, yet for thirty years previously they had been the object of the poor's suspicion and hatred. The poor would desperately need medical aid in 1832, yet their own attitudes, prejudices and mentalities were to drive them away from what little succour the medical profession could offer. At the root of this alienation was a consciousness that, far from being the friends of the people, the doctors were their enemies who preyed, for personal profit and success, on their helplessness and destitution. This process of alienation was gradual and spasmodic, stemming from the difficulties which the medical profession faced in obtaining an adequate supply of bodies on which medical students could practise the new science of morbid anatomy.

In order to progress medical science has frequently to act contrary to the instincts and prejudices of the public. At the present time vivisection and organ transplants raise serious moral and ethical problems. In the eighteenth and early nineteenth centuries popular protest resulted from the need to obtain bodies, the raw material for the new empirical teaching methods which had spread from the universities of Leyden and Edinburgh. The science of morbid anatomy, although of long-standing, only came to be accepted widely in the eighteenth century. Its increasing importance stimulated the growth of the independent medical schools which, although few in number at first, proliferated during the 1790s when trained surgeons for the forces were urgently required. Their numbers further increased after 1815 with the growing professionalisation of medicine until by 1832 there were seventeen private schools in London and fourteen in the provinces.[54]

Each student required three bodies on which to practise during his sixteen-month course in surgery and anatomy. By the 1820s, therefore, several thousand bodies were required per annum, but there was no legal provision for bodies on this scale.[55] The Murder Act of 1752, which ordered either public dissection or hanging in chains for executed murderers, failed to supply a quantity sufficient for the schools' needs. Surgeon-teachers came to rely on their own ingenuity to obtain the materials of their trade. Before the 1790s this usually led to small bands of students exhuming newly-buried corpses from cemeteries in the dead of night. As the demand for bodies intensified, however, the teachers became increasingly reliant on part-time bodysnatchers, who frequently combined their night-time activities with the respectable job of gravedigger, sexton or hospital porter. Exhuming bodies became a lucrative occupation. Ben Crouch, one-time leader of the notorious London Borough Gang, later agreed that body-snatching 'is worth following, if you can get subjects; a man may make a good living at it, if he is a sober man, and acts with judgement, and supplies the schools. . .'.[56]

Two gangs were to gain especial notoriety in London in the early nineteenth century. The first was Crouch's which was based in Southwark. Crouch was a powerful, bad-tempered, pock-marked individual with a weakness for exotic clothes. Like many other resurrectionists he had links with the London hospitals, his father having been a carpenter at Guy's. The gang included Joseph Butler, a 'short, good-tempered man with a laughing eye and Sancho Panza sort of expression', previously a porter at St Thomas.[57] Bill Hollis was a former sexton and Joseph Naples, who kept a diary of the gang's activities, was an ex-gravedigger. There was also the ex-prize fighter Bill Harnett, the dandified Jack Harnett and Tom Light, who had spent seven years in the hulks for stealing windows from coaches and was repeatedly being apprehended in the possession of stolen goods.[58]

Naples' diary graphically illustrates the gang's dissoluteness and debauchery. Frequently they were too drunk to rifle the graveyards. The following is an account of one week in their career.

Tuesday, 14 January 1812

At 1 a.m. got up, Bill Ben and me went to St Luke's, 2 adults; Jack, Dan Big Gates, 1 large and 1 small, took them to barthow. Came home and went to St Thomas', afterwards went to the other end of town for orders. At home all night.

Wednesday, 15th

Went to St Thomas's, Came back, pack'd up 2 large and 1 small for Edinburgh. At home all night.

Thursday, 16th

The party met at the Hatrichoak. Settled the above, Each man's share £8–4–7½d. At home all night.

Friday, 17th

Went and look out; came home wet at 11, party except Dan, went to hospital crib and got 4, was stopt by the patrols, Butler, Horse and Cart were taken.

Saturday, 18th

Went to the White Horse, Butler bailed: at home all night.

Sunday, 19th

Went and look'd out, at home all night, Could not get the horse out of the stable.

Monday, 20th

At home all day and night, Butler and Jack got drunk.

Tuesday, 21st

Look'd out, Jack and Butler drunk as before, hindered us going out. At home.

Wednesday, 22nd

At 4 o'clock in the morning got up, Bill and me went to the Hospital Crib and 1 for Mr Cooper's lectures, had a dispute with the party, at home all night. Ben got drunk.[59]

Sir Astley Cooper, the most eminent surgeon of his day, who perforce had to use the gang's services, called them 'the lowest dregs of degradation; I do not know that I can describe them better; there is no crime they would not commit, and as to myself, if they would imagine that I would make a good subject, they really would not have the smallest scruple, if they could do the thing undiscovered, to make a subject of me'.[60]

The gang disbanded in 1813, having dominated the body trade for a decade. Tom Light, having been repeatedly arrested, was jailed for pushing a cart containing seven bodies up Holborn Hill at 4.30 one February afternoon. He became a Methodist and was last seen leaving London with a newly-bought horse and cart. Crouch and Jack Harnett bought sutler's licences and pursued the British army through Spain, stripping bodies on the battlefields of their teeth. On returning to London they set up as false teeth dealers. Bill Harnett died of consumption in St

Thomas', begging not to be dissected, while Hollis died friendless and penniless after denouncing a horse thief who was hanged. Naples was to die of drink.[61]

In the 1820s Patrick Murphy gained a stranglehold on the body business. For a time he managed to double the price of bodies but his unscrupulous methods created such a furore that by the end of the decade it was virtually impossible to obtain bodies from graveyards. He would not countenance rival gangs; if they tried to undersell him, he

> burst in to the places in which bodies were contained, and spoiled them for dissection, and did not hesitate to commit barbarous acts for that purpose; or if there was a party of persons disposed to oppose him, he excited a riot against those individuals, and pointed them out as bad characters and resurrection men . . .[62]

He also made splendid examples of recalcitrant teachers. When Joshua Brookes of the Blenheim Street Private School refused to pay Murphy his customary douceur one year, decomposing bodies were left at either end of Blenheim Street. Two respectable women tripped over one and in the resulting uproar Brookes had to seek sanctuary in a nearby police station.

Owing to this adverse publicity it became increasingly difficult by the 1820s to raid the London cemeteries without being set upon by armed guards or falling foul of elaborately planned traps. An assortment of ingenious devices to deter graverobbing forced resurrectionists to travel further afield and adopt new stratagems. Some resorted to stealing bodies from houses and undertakers; others attended inquests on the unknown dead, claimed to be relatives and sold the body. Yet others took the sick to hospital and later returned to claim the body after death.[63] Such activities only further exposed the bodysnatchers to hostile public scrutiny.

There is no doubt that the poor hated resurrectionists, not just in London where they were well organised, but wherever the existence of a private anatomy school necessitated graverobbing. Their hatred was understandable. The same fundamentalist religious beliefs which made burial in unconsecrated ground unacceptable applied equally to resurrectionism. The doctrine of 'Resurrection of the Flesh' has been part of the basic faith of Western Christendom throughout the ages. It was incorporated in the Apostles' Creed; accepted by the Fourth Lateran Council; embodied in Anglican teaching via the Book of Homilies and Hooker's work; and taught in Calvin's Institutes and in Luther's small Catechism. The Early Fathers argued that the wicked could not receive their just deserts without the resurrection of the flesh. Justice demanded recompense in a future life; if applied only to the soul, justice could not be achieved.[64] In an age when the reading of the Bible was commonplace and its interpretation *personal*, such statements as 'the identical structure which death had previously destroyed' will be restored, or the 'particles composing each individual's flesh' will be collected together, were unambiguous and allowed of only one interpretation.[65]

In addition to the religious objections, the use of the body in anatomy theatres was regarded as morally degrading. The law permitted only the dissection of convicted murderers. To be dissected, therefore, carried a social stigma; it also denied a peaceful resting place to the poor. It was not as if they personally benefited from an improved system of medical education, except in the long term. Very few surgeons and doctors came into contact with the poor and apothecaries did not require certificates from anatomy schools to become qualified. The bodies of the poor were being used for the benefit of the wealthy, those who could pay medical fees. It is not surprising that Ben Crouch complained in 1828 that the poor 'would not mind shooting a man as dead as a robber, if they caught him in a churchyard; if you were pointed out that you were a resurrection man, they are very prejudiced against you'.[66]

The medical profession, those who employed the body-snatchers, were equally unpopular, particularly when it was shown that the surgeon-teachers had little respect for the dead bodies they used. In 1831, for example, the Aberdeen anatomy school was destroyed by a crowd after a dog was found wandering the streets with human bones which it had dug up from the school's backyard.[67] Student pranks also resulted in popular retribution. On one occasion in London a riot erupted after a student dropped a leg down the chimney of a house next door to the anatomy theatre. It fell into a pot of stew and gave a chimney-sweep's wife hysterics.[68] Such examples, and many more could be instanced from throughout the country, destroyed the medical profession's reputation in the eyes of the poor.

It was, however, a series of events between 1828 and 1831 which finally severed the links between the poor and medical practitioners. The first was the Select Committee of Inquiry into Anatomy, established in 1828 as the result of two judicial decisions in Lancashire which made it an offence for a medical man to have possession of a dead body, if it could be shown that he knew how the body had been obtained.[69] According to this legal interpretation, if a practitioner obtained a body on which to practise, he was committing a common law offence; if he made an error whilst operating, he could be sued by civil action. Two Lancashire judges had unwittingly jeopardised the future development of modern medical science.

The Committee of Inquiry was strongly influenced by Henry Warburton and Francis Place, both of whom belonged to that close-knit group of political economists who adhered to the ideas and philosophy of Jeremy Bentham. Inspired by the greatest happiness principle, the Committee's recommendations sacrificed the feelings of the poor for the greater good of a scientifically trained medical profession. Following the French example the Committee suggested that the bodies of those who during life had been maintained at public expense and who had died in workhouses, hospitals or other charitable institutions should, if not claimed by next of kin within a certain time of death, be given to an anatomist. In a classical espousal of the Theory of Utility they justified themselves by claiming that the misery of those related to the exhumed dead could only be diminished 'by giving up for dissection a certain portion of the whole, in order to preserve the remainder from disturbance'. Their report ended, 'To neglect the practice of dissection, would lead to the great aggravation of human misery; since anatomy, if not learned by that practice, must be learned by mangling the living.' The onus for keeping the medical schools running still lay with the poor, those least able to defend themselves both before and after death.

The Committee's final warning was prophetic, for only four months later the Burke and Hare outrages in Edinburgh were uncovered. Between December 1827 and October 1828 Burke and Hare murdered at least sixteen people and sold their bodies to Robert Knox of the independent medical school in Edinburgh. This scandal added a new dimension to popular attitudes to the medical profession. The fortuitous manner in which the murders had been discovered raised the possibility that these were not isolated phenomena. A great outcry followed and Knox was made a scapegoat, which a popular ballad confirmed:

Up the close and down the stair,
But and ben with Burke and Hare,
Burke's the butcher, Hare's the thief,
Knox the boy that buys the beef.[70]

At the same time a new word entered the English language, that of 'burking', defined as murdering by suffocation or murdering so as to produce few marks of violence with the motive of selling the corpses to the medical profession.

These revelations caused a wave of fear which swept the country. From Leeds, York, Kelso, Newcastle, Leicester, Glasgow, Nottingham, Balsall, Birmingham and Somers Town came reports of attempted or mock burkings. In Brighton people were reported to be afraid of walking the streets at night, because of a rumour that prowlers were waiting to slap plasters over victims' mouths. (There was no truth in the rumour, but a public dissection had recently taken place in Brighton.) In Barnet at this time, a grazier was found on his roof crying for help. He had dreamt that two men and a woman were planning to kill him and take his body to a hospital. Awakening, he had knocked a hole in the ceiling and climbed onto the roof, where he almost froze to death. Other reports were more sinister. In Nottingham a crowd set off in pursuit of a man suspected of decoying a young child away. The man escaped, but the crowd turned on a local quack doctor whom they believed to be implicated, attacked his house, broke his windows and if the police had not arrived, 'would probably have killed the occupier'.[71]

Many of these incidents occurred far away from schools of anatomy; nevertheless the same fears existed. This was partly owing to the rumour chain and partly to the fact that with bodies in short supply, resurrectionists were seeking victims ever further afield. Once the kernel of fear existed it easily grew into huge proportions, especially in a peripatetic society where people were frequently absent from their usual haunts. In the popular imagination they were soon regarded as victims of the burkers. Some of these fears were justified, for in 1831 three other gangs of burkers were arrested in London.[72] These revelations rekindled feelings of outrage and blind anger. They were more reprehensible in that the murderers were known resurrectionists, unlike Burke and Hare who had never exhumed bodies from cemeteries. Again, popular hatred was directed at the medical profession, although the apprehension of one group was due to the vigilance of Robert Grainger of the Webb Street School of Anatomy. The lesson of Edinburgh had not been learned and the syndrome had been repeated. The London burkers had taken their cue from Edinburgh as a means of revamping their trade when it was in depression. The medical authorities had again sought their own self-interest and took insufficient notice of the bodies which came into their possession.[73]

The London burking outrages occurred at the same time as cholera first reached Britain in the autumn of 1831. They caused yet another outbreak of fear and rumours, which coincided in time with cholera fears. Both sets of rumours and fears became enmeshed in one anti-doctor fear which saw the medical profession as a whole as antagonists. All became tarred with the same brush. This would explain the poison therapy which developed at the very beginning of the cholera epidemic. It was only a 'logical' rumour if the doctors had a motive for killing the poor and this the needs of dissection gave them.

An examination of the crowds' taunts and slogans during the disturbances reinforces this conclusion. In the first riot in Glasgow the doctors were called 'burkers'. Rioters in two of the London disturbances thought that cholera victims would be given to anatomy surgeons.[74] The slogan 'burker' was also used in Bristol and in three of the Liverpool disturbances, while accusations of murder were flung at doctors in Leeds, Sheffield and Manchester.[75] It was in Paisley in March and Manchester in September 1832, however, where the fears of resurrectionism and the fears of cholera were most closely interlinked. In both cases full-scale riots were the consequence.

Like many other towns at this time, Paisley had a new burial ground, ready to take the expected cholera victims from amongst the poorest classes. On 26 March boys playing near the cemetery found the stock-in-trade of bodysnatchers (small shovels and a hook) under a bridge. A crowd rushed to the burial ground and found several of the graves empty. Having pulled up all the stobs, they marched into town carrying an empty coffin. Stopped by the magistrates, a struggle occurred in which the coffin was broken. One of the larger pieces was carried off by the crowd, who stoned the police. One who was injured took refuge in a nearby house which was stoned and the windows broken. The crowd then made off into town where they attacked the houses of the local medical men. Ten in all were attacked; only one, belonging to a Mr Stewart, who was sceptical of cholera's existence, remained untouched. Meanwhile a magistrate had persuaded the crowd to bypass the cholera hospital, but the cholera cart was seized and dragged through the streets. After causing considerable damage in town, the crowd was stopped by a magistrate who seized what little was left of the cart. The majority of rioters began to drift away, but one group, led by chimneysweeps called Green and Walsh, had already back-tracked and were attacking the hospital. They broke all the windows, destroyed every moveable article and, according to one account, broke into the spirit store. In the assault, one patient was hit on the head by a stone and subsequently died.

In the meantime another group marched towards the county administration buildings, where they came face to face with the military and officers of the Renfrewshire militia. The troops soon dispersed the crowd, which consisted 'almost entirely of half-grown lads and Irishmen'. Fifteen people were arrested for riot. A subsequent investigation by special constables discovered that of the eighty bodies in the graveyard, only three were missing.[76]

The riots in Manchester on 2 September centred on the Swan Street cholera hospital. Opposition to the hospital had begun when cholera arrived in July and police had had to guard the hospital gates and the burial ground. The local board of health had also been forced to employ a man (in addition to the driver and bearers) to prevent bystanders from approaching the cholera cart as it took patients to hospital.[77] The simmering feelings against the hospital erupted into a massive riot when an Irishman called Hare visited his four-year-old grandson in the hospital. The old man had hoped to take his grandson home, for on the previous day he had been recovering rapidly. Hare, who was the boy's closest relative as the parents had died of cholera, was refused admittance. Having gone to complain to the board of health, he returned to discover that the boy was dead and already buried. The next day, Hare and his friends exhumed the body and found that the boy's head was missing, it having been replaced by a brick in the coffin. Immediately they marched towards the hospital, carrying the coffin aloft. A crowd, estimated at 3,000, collected behind the procession. 'The cries of execration against the doctors was very general and an almost unanimous shout of "To the hospital, pull it to the ground", took place.' In Oldham Street, a surgeon was forced to alight from his gig and inspect the body. Having agreed to the necessity of an inquiry, he was allowed to proceed on his journey. The crowd marched to the hospital, broke its windows, pulled down a surrounding wall and carried the sick home (some died shortly afterwards). Every moveable object in the hospital was destroyed and the new spring cholera carts burned. A cutless-wielding band of policemen arrived who had to defend their own lock-ups from the crowd's attacks. Eventually four troops of hussars arrived with a magistrate, who threatened to read the Riot Act. With the help of a Roman Catholic priest the crowd calmed down, although nine people were arrested. One section of the crowd moved off towards Piccadilly with the coffin but were eventually stopped by the police who arrested a further three rioters.

At a subsequent inquiry it was found that a surgeon called Robert Oldham had bribed the boy's Irish nurse and had decapitated the body in the hospital. Oldham fled and although a warrant was issued for his arrest he seems to have successfully disappeared. The twelve arrested rioters, nearly all of whom were Irish, went before a magistrate who discharged four and bailed the rest at £20 to attend the next sessions.[78]

The two most serious riots, therefore, those which required the use of troops, were stimulated by the connection of anti-anatomy and cholera fears in the popular mind. Popular attitudes towards cholera were grafted onto an already existing mistrust and hatred of the medical profession. All the anti-doctor riots were fuelled by the same legitimising notions. As Edward Thompson has shown in relation to food riots, the poor felt they had a moral right to redress grievances by direct action when lawful authority gave them no protection.[79] Indeed, at this very time, the law regarding dissection was being altered, against the poor's interest, for Henry Warburton had just successfully steered his second Anatomy Bill, which was based on the recommendations of the 1828 Committee of Inquiry, through a largely indifferent House of Commons. The Bill had been extremely unpopular (it was called the Dead Body Bill by the poor). Francis Place, himself a firm adherent of the Bill, wrote that 'the feelings of nearly the whole people were averse to any interference of the legislature, unless it should be, perhaps, to hang all resurrection-men'.[80]

With the law no deterrent, the poor took matters into their own hands and administered their own form of rough social justice. Before 1832 this usually took the form of physically assaulting resurrectionists and doctors and attacking schools of anatomy. In 1828, for example, four bodysnatchers were pursued from St James' churchyard in Clerkenwell by the Watch and some Irish skindressers. They took refuge in the Fleet Ditch but were dragged out 'by the indignant multitude, apparently thirsting to imbue their hands in the blood of these unfortunate wretches'. One was so seriously injured that he was taken immediately to hospital. One of the skindressers was eventually fined 50 shillings for assaulting a bodysnatcher as he was being taken to court.[81]

Similar reactions were in evidence in Edinburgh a few years previously, when a coach carrying an empty coffin was stopped by a crowd. The police managed to save the driver, but the coach was driven through the streets, overturned, smashed and burned, the crowd dancing gleefully around the bonfire. At about the same date, two Americans visiting Linlithgow Abbey at nightfall were mistaken for resurrectionists and assaulted.[82]

The recent London burkings and the introduction of Warburton's Bill in Parliament kept the anatomy issue alive during the cholera epidemic. Other, more local events, heightened public awareness in some of the areas where cholera disturbances took place. At 6 a.m. one morning in April 1832, for example, a policeman stopped a cart carrying three men in the New Cross Road heading towards London. On searching the cart he found hidden under some rubbish two naked bodies. The men were arrested and taken to the local police station, around which a huge crowd (estimated at 2,000 by the over-zealous *Times*) gathered. Forty policemen were required to take the prisoners to Deptford magistrate's court, many of whom were injured by flying stones, brickbats and mud.[83]

Discoveries of bodysnatchers recently having been at work occurred elsewhere also. All took place before the cholera reached each particular town. In Leeds a gang of bodysnatchers were arrested for stealing a body in November 1831; in Liverpool a gang was at work in the spring of 1832. The activities of resurrectionists in Stoke Damerell churchyard were still fresh in people's minds in the South-West when the cholera arrived.[84] All were reported in local newspapers and helped to keep feelings high.

The result was that when cholera arrived and special hospitals were established, any rumour which developed could be integrated into an already existing worldview. Consequently, direct action during the epidemic was similar to that which had occurred when resurrectionists were assaulted in the 1820s. Specific targets were always attacked and there is little evidence that the rioters took the opportunity of indulging in general destruction (a library destroyed in Paisley was next door to a doctor's house). When considerable damage to property was effected, as in Paisley, Manchester, Aberdeen and Sheffield (in 1835), the poor were always impelled by some legitimising notion. Because, however, action was usually the result of rumours, some preposterous events have been recorded. In April 1831, for example, a crowd attacked a house in Manchester and almost killed the inmates, after a rumour spread that a woman was kidnapping children to use as filling for veal pies. While the popular story of Sweeney Todd may have influenced the crowd, it is also true that the preparer of bodies at the local school of anatomy lodged at the house and this was sufficient, given the prevailing public mood, for direct action to be taken.[85] Similarly in Dumfries in November 1832, the poor attempted to catch and assault a Mr Green, whom they blamed for bringing cholera to the town. He had given a demonstration of his hot air balloon just before cholera broke out and was subsequently accused of bringing the disease back to earth with him. Given the circumstances, the 'logic' was reasonable, especially when atmospheric theories of disease causation were popular. (Most likely, of course, one of the visitors who came to see the show brought cholera with him.)[86]

The victims of the crowds' vengeance were also carefully selected. Very few innocent people were deliberately attacked—

in the eyes of the poor the medical profession was guilty of course. However, relatives, friends and colleagues of the suspected were sometimes found guilty by association. The consorts of Burke and Hare, for example, were attacked and Burke's brother lost his job as a scavenger and given money to leave Edinburgh before he suffered popular retribution. The unfortunate woman assaulted on leaving the Liverpool cholera hospital in April 1832 is another example, while 'innocent' cholera cart attendants were also attacked.

Behind the expressions of discontent reflected in the cholera disturbances of 1832 there existed a desire amongst the poor to demand social justice. Cholera was assimilated into a worldview which perceived a threat to the whole complex nexus of traditional values and beliefs of a culture existing outside the bounds of respectable society. As such, cholera was just one further threat to the 'culture of poverty'. On its own, it caused fear and temporary blind panic, which found expression in the shunning of victims and their relatives. But when the dominant culture intervened, as with the Anatomy Bill or the burial regulations, the clash of cultures resulted in direct action whenever a precipitating incident sparked it off. The chief scapegoats were the medical profession, but they were more than just surrogates or the only representatives of the dominant culture readily available for attack. They had most to gain from an abundant supply of dead poor. This would explain why the poison theory, universally believed in Europe in 1831 and 1832, was given a different emphasis in Britain. In France it was believed that the doctors were murdering the poor *on behalf of the rich.*[87] To do this effectively, water supplies had to be polluted with poison. In St Petersburg, foreign doctors were the scapegoats, while in subsequent riots in the Russian military colonies, the doctors were believed to be involved with the military chiefs in a conspiracy to diminish the total population, the colonies being overcrowded.[88] In Hungary, the nobility had bribed quarantine officers and doctors to poison the peasantry by polluting wells with what turned out to be chlorate of lime.[89]

Prevailing social tensions, therefore, moulded the poison theory to suit prevailing conditions. From the evidence available, the conspiracies on a wide scale, which are such a feature of European response to cholera, did not exist in Britain. The medical profession was accused only of murdering individual patients; wholesale slaughter of the poor was not the aim, but an adequate supply of bodies for dissection. In only one disturbance were gentlemen implicated in murder and that was in Bristol, where burial grounds and St Peter's Hospital—the local poorhouse, bedlam and vagrant house—were the foci of unrest. One rumour circulating was that 'gentlemen' were suffocating the poor to be rid of them. These were obviously meant to be the poorhouse authorities, who at this time were beset by the problem of overcrowding, having 600 inmates with facilities for only 300.[90]

With this one possible exception, where fears were generated similar to those in the Russian military colonies, cholera fears in Britain in 1832 were not expressed in terms of a major conspiracy by one class against another. Thus, while the class theories of Chevalier and Baehrel are, in general terms, substantiated by British evidence, tension in Britain could find a precise, particular and narrow focus, which made the popular cholera actions less 'global' in their significance. The traditional enemy was dealt with in a traditional and 'legitimate' manner. In the same way that bread rioters legitimised themselves by marching behind a loaf stuck on a pike, the anatomy and cholera rioters frequently marched with their own emblem. When resurrectionists stole Dick Turpin's body in York in 1739, a crowd pursued them and found the body in a surgeon's garden. They carried it through town on a board in a triumphal manner and later buried it in unslaked lime.[91] In Paisley the crowd carried first a coffin and then the cholera cart before them as emblems. In Manchester they carried the body of the young boy through town. These were emblems which symbolised the victory of popular morality and society's inequalities in an age when the law failed to give the poor adequate protection.

8

The People and the Cholera: (ii) The Cholera in Social and Political Context

THE preceding chapter has focused on the essentially specific and local stimuli which conditioned popular motivation and generated hostile outbursts of a *traditional* nature. It is necessary now to broaden the context and consider why the cholera disturbances were not subsumed into the general unrest of the period and did not, as in Europe, accentuate class feelings. After all, the disturbances did not occur in a vacuum but during a period of acute political and industrial unrest. Indeed, Eversley has argued that cholera coincided, 'et pas entièrement par hasard, avec une période d'agitation généralisée; le sort de la Réforme électorale était alors incertain et la situation politique se trouvait de ce fait aggravée'.[1] Such was the close relationship between cholera and reform, he felt, that the reduction of the cholera fear was mostly due to the calming of political tension following the passing of the Reform Bill.

This relationship, superficially attractive, collapses when the period is analysed closely, for the crisis periods of reform, October 1831 and May 1832, do not synchronise with the crisis periods of cholera in the major towns. In October, cholera was present only in Sunderland and had not yet been officially confirmed. Rumours and fears existed, but there were no demonstrations. Similarly, in May 1832 cholera had fortunately but definitely deserted London and had not yet infected any of the English towns where there were to be cholera riots. Liverpool was infected on 1 June (one isolated case had occurred on 17 May), Leeds on 29 May, Manchester on 29 June, and Birmingham, Sheffield, Bristol and Exeter in July.[2] Of the Scottish towns, Edinburgh, Glasgow and Paisley were infected during a lull in the Reform Bill proceedings, while Dumfries' epidemic began in November 1832. Almost all the disturbances, therefore, occurred after the Reform Bill became law. It is feasible, of course, that the passing of the Bill *increased* tension; if the poor misguidedly believed that they had been given the vote, a cull of their numbers, in the guise of a new disease, could be viewed as one way in which the ruling classes attempted to retain political power. Yet there is no evidence to suggest that such a rationalisation, which would have been comparable with beliefs held in eastern Europe in 1831, played any part in generating disturbances in Britain in 1832.

Nor is there any real evidence to suggest that fear of cholera exerted any influence during the industrial disturbances of this period. Again, lack of synchronisation is the key. Newcastle, for example, was suffering from high unemployment, acute distress, strikes and an epidemic at about the same time, yet there were no disturbances motivated by cholera, even in the colliery villages where striking miners were evicted from their tied homes while the disease raged. Similarly, industrial disturbances occurring in Bilston in December 1831 were followed by high unemployment in 1832. The Bilston epidemic was to be one of the worst in the country, with 2,250 cases and 693 deaths from a population of 14,500, but no disturbances erupted there.[3] Although it is true, therefore, that political or industrial unrest existed in towns where there were to be cholera disturbances, there were other towns which had these 'pre-conditions' and a major epidemic, yet failed to suffer from rioting. What distinguished the towns affected by cholera disturbances were not socio-economic conditions or political agitation so much as the presence of schools of anatomy. Of all the English towns which possessed private schools, only Hull and Newcastle failed to undergo some specific disturbance during the epidemic.

To understand why the cholera agitations remained separate from, or at least failed to be subsumed into, the general unrest in 1832, one must examine how the epidemic was used by the radicals in their battle for political reform. If any groups were to have influence over the poor it would be these, who articulated working-class feelings and acted on major channels for the transmission of political ideas to the masses. For English radicalism the years 1830 to 1832 were the climax of the battle between Old Corruption and Reform. While the radical leadership was divided on the merits of the particular scheme of reform put forward by the Whigs, on one issue at least they were united—the necessity of generating mass support for reform. Radical ideas could be effective only if they were given a mass base. To achieve this end the radical leaders had to convince the rank and file that society required fundamental alteration.[4] In this context cholera could have been of vital importance, for the radicals could have used it to highlight the contradictions and inequalities of that society.

But the reform movement was divided in 1832 on the question of whether or not to accept help from the middle-classes. To a considerable extent a radical's views on cholera were dependent on his particular allegiance at the time. Both middle-class and working-class radicals had their own strategies and tactical ploys which conditioned reactions to subjects having possible political repercussions. The middle-class radicals were primarily concerned with the passing of the Reform Bill. They were moderate reformers, to the left of the Whig party in general but including more radical reformers such as Francis Place, James Mill and Joseph Hume in London (all of whom were Benthamites and political economists), and Thomas Attwood and Joseph Parkes in Birmingham. Place and his colleagues represented and dominated the National Political Union and the Birmingham Political Union, through which they tried to unite middle- and working-class opinion in a drive to force the Whigs into passing as comprehensive a measure of reform as possible.[5]

Essentially, radicals of this ilk held middle-class norms and values. They were above all 'respectable', adhering to the middle-class values expressed in the works of Ricardo, Malthus and Bentham. They implicitly accepted the middle-class distinction between the deserving and undeserving poor.[6] Above all, they were law-abiding. This at first sight appears surprising, for during the Reform Bill agitation Place oscillated between warning the government of possible revolution and actually threatening it himself. But a strong case had been made to show that the rhetoric of the political unions in 1831 and 1832 was no more than a bluff to cajole the Whigs into passing the Reform Bill. It was a policy which Joseph Hamburger has called 'the language of menace'. James Mill was the instigator of this strategy.

> Mill visualised the ruler as conceding to a threat of revolution; for, as a rational being he would yield to the threat rather than follow the more costly procedure of resisting it. If these tactics were to be used successfully, it was necessary that the ruler really believe that revolution threaten . . . Mill's tactics required . . . that public feelings be formulated and interpreted in a portentous, even a threatening way, and the public and especially the government, be persuaded that this appearance corresponded to the reality. The emphasis was placed on appearances.[7]

While Hamburger overestimates the role Mill played in agitation at this time and underrates the deep-seated unrest in the country itself, especially in October 1831 and May 1832, his analysis does raise the question of how Mill and Place in London and Parkes in Birmingham should have used the threat of cholera within the confines of their overall strategy. The knowledge of uprisings in eastern Europe could have been used as a lever to spur on the Whigs to pass the Bill before cholera, with its threat of social upheaval, arrived. But the middle-class radicals were seemingly unwilling to use cholera as a weapon against the ministry. Indeed, they saw the prospect of cholera being used as a weapon against themselves. In December 1831, when cholera was confined to the North-East, Place wrote to Hume,

> The cholera will spread all over the country, and by the time the Bill shall have reached the Third Reading, and the country shall have become tired, if not wearied out and disgusted, we shall have quarantine regulations against our shipping in all parts of the world. The consequences may be a great impediment to navigation, diminution of trade and commerce, embarrassment, stagnation, panic, multitudes of people discharged in all our great manufactures.[8]

Cholera was therefore seen as a threat, able to upset the momentum for reform in three ways. First, the government's commercial restrictions could alienate that very sector of society which Place and his colleagues were manipulating as the major supporters of the government outside Parliament. Second, the possible unemployment following quarantine's implementation might lead to serious industrial disturbances. This would be real unrest, not the *ersatz* variety of the middle-class radicals. Third, cholera might be used by the Tories as a tool to divert attention away from the Reform Bill.

To fully appreciate the middle-class radicals' view on cholera in late 1831 it is necessary to deal with the political situation in some detail. The second Reform Bill had been thrown out by the Lords on 8 October and was followed in the next few weeks by increasing unrest, culminating in the major riots in Bristol, Nottingham and Derby. Disillusioned by the failure of their Bill and alarmed by the rioting, the Whigs decided not to recall Parliament until January 1832. In the meantime they entered into negotiations with the Tories to find ways of compromising on the Reform Bill.[9] Such a policy was anathema to the radicals and smacked of treason. As a protest movement calling for the immediate reintroduction of the Reform Bill burgeoned in London, the government ordered in troops and swore in special constables. Fortunately, negotiations with the Tories broke down and on 22 November it was decided to reconvene Parliament on 6 December. Immediately, according to Place, 'The people became calm, and agitation in most places ceased.'[10]

The middle-class radicals' position on cholera must be seen in the light of this political background. A Whig-Tory alliance was a possibility, which would be formed at the radicals' expense. To achieve their aims, the Tories were prepared to use every weapon available, including the threat of cholera. Evidence from *The Examiner* shows that the middle-class radicals took this prospect seriously. It was vital, therefore, that cholera be shown to be a Tory hoax, a humbug, used as a vehicle to spread alarm. That some Tories saw the disease in this light is true. Sir Edward Sugden, former Solicitor General in the last Tory administration, was reported to have said that cholera 'will be serviceable as a diversion'.[11] Robert Ferguson's scaremongering article in the *Quarterly Review* was also seen as representing Tory opinion and tactics, deliberately creating a climate of panic.

> Between the plague of the House of Lords and the pestilence, the public mind has been kept in a seasonable horror this grim month. If one alarm subsides, another immediately springs up. If the accounts from Sunderland are more favourable, the

> reports from Brighton are 'such as to excite the most serious apprehensions'. If the cholera remits, the Cumberland influence, the epityrannic, instantly becomes ascendant. If our bowels seem for a moment safe, the frame of society is threatened with convulsion; if health improves, the Constitution falls into danger! Scarcely have we thanked Heaven that our stores from the Apothecary, the laudanum, the opium, the calomel, the capsicum, are likely to be useless, when we are advised to lay in munitions of war against the Boroughmongers—or, in default of fear of them, a pauper rebellion is threatened. Fright is the order of the day.[12]

Fear of cholera, therefore, neatly dovetailed with fear of reform. To overcome the latter, the middle-class radicals had to destroy the former. To do this they used the weapons of satire and advanced medical theory. *The Examiner*, for example, quoted with approval a placard in a grocer's shopwindow in Gray's Inn Lane which suggested that the best way of escaping cholera was 'to avoid by all possible means any communication or connexion with anti-reformers'. It also parodied the prayers issued by the Anglican Church against cholera, to suggest the Tory-cholera link.

With one accord, let all the Outs their
joyful voices raise,
And sing unto the Lords a song of wonder,
love and praise;
To them be praise, whose wise delays have
staved off the intolerable measures of
Reform, till folks are frightened by the
cholera.

Oh, the cholera,
The sweet spasmodic cholera!
Last prop of power legitimate, the kind,
convenient cholera!

All men of nauseating mouths and giddy at
the head,
E.G., all civic speakers must be soundly
boiled and bled;

There shan't be heard another word of
England's rights or wrongs,
We'll clap 'em in an iron cage, and feed
'em with the tongs.

Oh, the cholera!
For certain 'tis the cholera.
Off with 'em to the Station House—the
rogues have got the cholera.[13]

Satire was supported by the more reasoned arguments of Edwin Chadwick, who was responsible for most of the articles on cholera in *The Examiner*. Chadwick, who believed that cholera was not a new disease but a variation of an old one, was hostile to the Central Board of Health, because of their contagionist philosophy and because their failure to insist on the accumulation of accurate statistics in Sunderland had increased unnecessary alarm. A comparison between cholera and typhus data would have shown, thought Chadwick, that the latter was more fatal.[14] His whole policy was aimed at reducing fear and consternation and at attacking the contagionist ideology prevalent amongst the medical elite. 'There are no people such fools in medicine as the fools of quality. An intelligent Board of Health would have been of great service; but a job has been driven even against a pestilence.'[15]

There can be little doubt that Chadwick was swayed by the ideas of Thomas Southwood Smith at this time, for they had known each other (and Neil Arnott) since 1824.[16] Smith believed in a unitary view of fever, which ran contrary to the growing trend amongst the British medical profession towards an acceptance of disease specificity, and Chadwick swallowed this theory whole. Personal conviction, therefore, played some part in explaining his noncontagionist arguments in 1831–32, yet they also offered several advantages to the middle-class radicals. First, the noncontagionist position minimised the unknown aspect of cholera, which could now be seen as an indigenous disease in a new guise. Second, by showing that cholera was dependent on local conditions for virulence and spread, it reduced the prospect of panic caused by fear of cholera's rapid and indiscriminate diffusion. Third, it was obviously futile to continue with quarantine regulations if the disease had originated within the country.

It was this last argument which the radicals dwelt on after December 1831. For once the government introduced the third Reform Bill, cholera as a threat to the radicals' political ambitions disappeared. No longer could it be used by the Tories as a powerful delaying factor. It became a temporary issue again in February 1832 when cholera struck London itself, but the swiftness with which the Cholera Prevention Act was passed, and the arguments of the medically trained Joseph Hume in Parliament, prevented any call for a prorogation. (Hume's belief in cholera's noncontagiousness did not, however, prevent him from cancelling a meeting in cholera-infected Limehouse in February at which he was to be guest speaker.)[17]

During the crisis of the Days of May cholera had disappeared from London and from most of the country and was not therefore a threat. It did not prevent, for instance, the monster meetings which the radicals used to exert extra-parliamentary pressure on the king and Wellington. By this time the middle-class radicals had reverted to seeing cholera from the standpoint of strict political economists. Cholera was still a hoax, not on the part of the Tories, but on the part of the reactionary medical profession abetted by the government, aimed at usurping people's natural rights and at allowing medical vendors and jobbers at the parish and government level to make a handsome profit.[18] Contagionism attacked the foundations of political economy. It unnecessarily interfered with trade, gave increased power to the parochial authorities (including the select vestries against which the radicals had been waging war), and increased public expenditure.

In 1832, therefore, the object of middle-class radical attack moved from the concept of cholera as an anti-reform tool to the Old Corruption philosophy behind Central Board of Health activity. Cholera was still a humbug, but no longer a disease hatched in the fertile mind of a Tory. The middle-class radicals never saw cholera as more than an unwelcome weapon in the opposition's armoury. It was a mere irritation which temporarily divided attention with the main issue, the question of reform.

Amongst the working-class radicals in 1832 cholera was taken more seriously. Working-class radicalism centred around the

National Union of the Working Classes in London and the manhood suffrage Political Unions in the Northern and Midland manufacturing areas which were not influenced by the middle-classes and were Painite in inspiration. The London leaders were Hetherington, Watson, Cleave, Benbow and Lovett. Although they were in contact with working-class radicals in the North, they were never to be as well organised as the NPU and BPU.[19] In London they were not even united on some essential points of their programme. While most of them opposed the Reform Bill as a betrayal of the radical movement some, for example, William Carpenter, Thomas Wakley and Cobbett, came to see the Reform Bill as the necessary first step towards universal manhood suffrage.[20] The methods proposed to achieve their aims covered a wide spectrum, from the moderate tendencies of Watson and Hetherington to the revolutionary plans of Benbow, who sought mass agitation and confrontation.[21] Place was being less than just when he wrote, 'The great peculiarity causing a difference between the Political Unions and the Unions of the working classes was that the first desired the reform bill to prevent a revolution, the last desired its destruction as a means of producing a revolution.'[22] But the working-class radicals were united in their adherence to a political solution to social ills and in a belief in the traditional radical Painite programme.

Amongst this rather heterogeneous group, it was the individualists who regarded cholera as a humbug. Carlile, egotistically opposed to the NUWC ('I have nothing to do with any association, and do not seek . . . assistance from anything of the kind'),[23] saw cholera as a job. Incarcerated in Giltspur Street Compter in July 1832 he pointed to the cynicism of the authorities who wooed cholera before it came but who on its appearance (he alluded to its second outbreak in London) did nothing but thank God that it had disappeared.[24] Cobbett, a believer in the Reform Bill (half a loaf was better than none), saw cholera as a threat to personal liberty, for the powers of the Cholera Act were theoretically unlimited. Precautionary measures only signified that the rich feared the effects of contagion from the poor (he noted that the 'chopsticks' in Norfolk called the blankets given out by the local boards 'scareblankets').[25] Cobbett, who was apparently the first to coin the phrase 'cholera humbug', saw cholera as one further way in which the rich could frighten the poor into submission. *The Examiner* reported a conversation Cobbett supposedly had with a Hampshire man:

> *Hampshire man:* And this cholera morbus sir, don't you think it's a sort of shohoy to frighten us out of reform?
> *Cobbett:* Not exactly that, but when one of your children has got the hick-ups . . .
> *Hampshire Man:* Aye, then my dame tells it some frightful lie, and away goes the hick-ups.
> *Cobbett:* Just so.
> *Hampshire Man:* Aye, but they won't frighten us with their cholera morbus, and make us contented with potatoes and water.[26]

Carlile and Cobbett were the only major working-class leaders in London to see cholera as a humbug. Eversley has suggested that Cobbett, if not the writer, was the inspiration for a poster placarded around Lambeth in February 1832 which suggested that,

> A set of half-starved doctors, apothecaries' clerks, and jobbers in parish funds have endeavoured to frighten the nation into a lavish expenditure; with the government they have succeeded in carrying a Bill that will afford rich pickings . . .[27]

Their other allies in promoting the cholera humbug were the satirical journals *The Devil in London* and *Figaro in London*, both of which were only on the fringes of the campaign for a free and unstamped press.

For the majority of the working-class radicals, however, cholera was no humbug, especially once it began to spread rapidly in June and July. It may have been used to enrich some of the medical profession, yet it was real, one more example of an inequitable society.[28] When cholera first broke out in London, Hetherington wrote,

> The cholera has arrived amongst us, and this, among other blessings, we have to lay at the door of our 'glorious constitution', for it is a disease begotten of that poverty and wretchedness which are occasioned by the wealth and luxury of the few to whom only the constitution belongs.[29]

An unequal society was thus the cause of cholera. This etiological decision was made on the basis of concrete and easily observable evidence: the squalid conditions in the London parishes. Indignation was rightly aroused by the state of Spitalfields, where the common picture of poverty, overcrowding and insanitary living conditions was exposed by the *Poor Man's Guardian* in February. Of all the social groups which 'discovered' working class poverty during the epidemic, the working class radicals most clearly identified themselves with the poor. At the same time as the *Guardian* was showing shock and horror, Thomas Wakley in *The Lancet* was fulminating against the medical profession for not publicising the abominable conditions in which the poor lived.[30]

Yet the remedies which the radicals offered were of only marginal utility. They advised temperance and moderation, classic official and middle-class doctrine. Under the heading 'Useful Knowledge for Gin-Drinkers and Smokers', Hetherington reprinted from the *Morning Herald* a letter which attempted to prove that most of the Sunderland cholera victims were drink and smoke addicts.[31] According to George Jacob Holyoake, Hetherington himself firmly believed in temperance as a cholera preventative: he was to find to his cost in 1849 that he was mistaken, for it was to be cholera which killed him.[32] Excessive drinking, however, was rightly seen by the radicals as a major obstacle to their overall aims. Later in the year James Lorymer claimed that the September cholera riot in Manchester demonstrated the people's unreadiness for universal suffrage. The main hindrance was cheap gin, which was sold in nearly a thousand gin shops in Manchester alone. 'Unless political knowledge is rendered cheaper than gin etc, riots and rows, more disturbances without any salutary object in view, may be expected. . . . The government consequently, is the remote cause of all riots similar to the cholera riot at Manchester.'[33]

If the call for temperance smacked of the imposition of the dominant culture, the other radical solution was more in keeping with their traditional programme. They demanded that the poor should, of right, be given the means to alleviate poverty and thereby strike at the root of cholera. But so outraged were the radicals by the scenes of misery that they had witnessed that they came close to counselling insurrection.

> You must endure your present state of wretchedness no longer, you are reduced to the last stage of misery; you have no other alternative left—either effectual relief or death, and better at once perish in the attempt to work the salvation of yourselves and your posterity, than tamely endure the agony of the fatal cholera. . . . Rather than endure [your sufferings] longer you had better at once provoke the bayonets of tyranny to put a speedy termination to them.[34]

Much of this was mere rhetoric, for few of the radicals were prepared to countenance that type of insurrection. In the aftermath of the Bristol riots, for instance, Lovett told Melbourne that far from seeking a similar uprising in London, the NUWC members were prepared to be sworn in as special constables to preserve public order.[35] In April 1832 Lovett, Cleave and Osborne, replying to Hume's query in *The Examiner* as to what the NUWC would do if the Reform Bill were again rejected, wrote that

> We do not suppose anything; but feeling that an odious oligarchy (in which we include 'Whigs and Tories') have enslaved the many, we are prepared to act with the greater number for the general good, whenever an opportunity presents itself as the most likely to secure to the people their undoubted rights; in case the Bill be rejected a second time, we hope the Union and its friends 'will stand at ease'.[36]

The 'people' here alluded to were not, however, the mob or the dangerous classes. In November 1831 Cleave admitted that London had a mob similar to the one in Bristol, but it had no dealings with the NUWC. The Bristol rioters were 'the scum and refuse of an accursed system, which was now happily crumbling to pieces'.[37] Cleave, and Lorymer for that matter, were implicitly distinguishing between the deserving and the undeserving poor. The former were the hard-working, persevering labouring poor; the latter were the incorrigibles, idle yet reckless enough seriously to compromise the delicate position of the NUWC. There was then a tension in the working-class radicals' analysis of cholera. Cholera was indeed symptomatic of a society moulded by Old Corruption. Everyone suffered from its effects but the poorest suffered most. Yet it was this stratum of society which the NUWC could not, and did not want to, reach.

This was demonstrated by the NUWC's decision to turn the Fast Day of 21 March 1832 into a Day of Farce. The idea of a day of fasting, aimed at propitiating the Almighty, was suggested in Parliament by Percival, the deranged Irvingite. Amidst great embarrassment and the enthusiasm of the bishops, 21 March was set as the day of atonement. For the working-class radicals this was the height of hypocrisy. Poverty caused cholera and poverty resulted from the pernicious social system which enabled the few to live well at the expense of the many. To fast meant to go without meat; how could the poor fast when they so rarely ate meat even at the best of times? The poor should, therefore, ridicule the occasion and take advantage of the cheap meat which was bound to be available.[38]

It was James Watson who first suggested the opportunities for propaganda which the Fast Day presented. It was a chance 'to make a display, not only of their numbers, but of their destitution, peaceably but publicly. He deprecated all violence as the conduct of a mob and not of thoughtful and sensible men'.[39] In his pamphlet published in May 1832 Watson expanded on this:

> It was to express our contempt not only for the imbecility and bigotry of the individual who urged upon the government the appointment of a general fast, but also to manifest our hatred of hypocrisy, believing, as we conscientiously did, that a man like 'Lord Brougham' could never bring his mind to believe that the farce of a day being set apart for a general fast could produce any change in the decrees of Omnipotence. We had another object in view. We wished to let our tyrants and oppressors see that we felt and hated their oppression. We wished to give this peaceable expression to the feelings of our fellow-countrymen.[40]

The emphasis was on a peaceable demonstration of solidarity, responsibility and respectability. As meetings and marches were forbidden on public holidays, the NUWC decided to take a 'pre-lunch stroll'.[41] Every precaution was taken to prevent possible violence but everybody, including the 'ragamuffins' of the metropolis were invited to attend, the only requirement being that they remained sober. Those who felt unable to comply were asked to keep away.[42]

The NUWC's scheme was political: they intended to use the poor and destitute as an example of a political system which was cruel and unjust. Cholera was not the object of attack, but the government's reactions to the disease were. No short-term policy of alleviation was contemplated by the radicals; long-term aims predominated. Change the basis of society through political reform and the conditions which had caused cholera would disappear. It was hoped that the organised marching of the poor would shame 'the saintly hypocrites' on their way to attend religious services.[43] The marchers would then disperse and the NUWC members would be treated to a 'feast' at their respective classes. Those *members* who could not afford the meal would be subsidised by the remainder. No plans were made for the ragamuffins; they presumably were expected to return to their lairs.

Not surprisingly, the plans were misunderstood. Rumours circulated that the radicals were going to feed the poor and when the NUWC met in Finsbury Square on 21 March, there were, in addition to 20,000 members, another 100,000 present.[44] Their ultimate objective was Hyde Park and at 11 a.m. the march began. Their route, however, was barred at several places by squads of police. The authorities had over-reacted and 4,000 policemen and special constables had been quartered in various parts of London. Some were armed with cutlasses similar to the knives used by pork butchers and knackers. 'They are adopted to close fighting, such as boarding in a naval action.'[45] Keeping their tempers in a remarkable display of self-restraint and solidarity, the marchers twisted and turned through the streets of the City and Central London, until at Howland Street, near Tottenham Court Road, the police again stopped the procession, cutting the leaders off from the rank and file. Benbow lost his temper and a scuffle developed which resulted in several police injuries and seven arrests. The procession then broke up and the NUWC members returned to their classes, where they partook of 'a plain and substantial dinner', heard several excellent speeches, toasted 'Equal rights, which will supersede the necessity of either general or partial fasts', and listened to music.[46] Meanwhile, a crowd of 1,500 men, women and children, carrying baskets 'in expectation that there would be a giving out of food on the part of the Unions', were being dispersed from Finsbury Square by the police. The poor had been deserted. 'Their misfortune was laughed at by some and pitied by others. They cursed Saint Percival and the Unions also.'[47]

The 21 March was meant to be a symbolic day, when the distress caused by an iniquitous political system would be shown to the world. It was an attempt to lift the curtain behind which the poor lay and bring a beam of light and hope into their murky world. But it was transient and meant to be so. It was to last only as long as it took a hundred thousand people to walk from Finsbury Square to Hyde Park. The symbolism lay elsewhere. The poor had turned up in their droves because not even out-paupers were cared for on the Fast Day. In St Margaret's Westminster, for example, out-paupers were given a small piece of bread and cheese to last the day. A stonemason and his wife and six children was given six ounces of bread and one ounce of cheese, worth 1½d.[48] For the poor a compulsory day from work was serious, upsetting their hand-to-mouth existence. It virtually forced them to enter into the spirit of the Fast Day. But it was just this practical aspect which the working-class radicals failed to appreciate. When Benbow, Lovett, Watson and Osborne were tried for their part in the Fast Day riots, they dissociated themselves from the others arrested, suggesting they were tools of the Police Commissioner.[49] They had in fact been arrested in Finsbury Square when the police came to clear the streets. Of the six arrested with the procession in Tottenham Court Road of whom there is evidence, three were journeymen (an unemployed baker, a woodcutter and a carpenter); one an unemployed gentleman's servant; one a dock labourer; and one a master painter. All were found guilty of hurling missiles at the police. If not encouraged by the NUWC to act thus, it was Benbow's intransigence which had stimulated them. They were all fined £5; the NUWC leaders were acquitted. It took a small group of tradesmen, artisans and others, using Halfway House in Webber Street, to appreciate what the Fast Day really meant to the poor. There they distributed to each person with a ticket ten to twelve ounces of boiled beef or mutton, potatoes, bread and soup. Three hundred were thus fed.[50] This may well have smacked of charity, but for the poor the needs of the day outweighed the visions of the future.

Thus neither the NPU nor the NUWC identified themselves with the poor in their struggle against cholera. Both leaderships re-orientated the disease to marry it with their own pressing *political* considerations. For the basically apolitical poor this was insufficient. Although the NUWC was stumbling towards an awareness of cholera as an indicator of social inequality, the National Farce Day must be seen more as an indictment of Old Corruption than as an attack on social inequality *per se*.

The radicals' failure to take the social lesson of cholera can partly be explained by their attitude to 'the People'. Without doubt the working-class radicals felt an affinity with the mass of the population, but their appeal to the masses fell on deaf ears, or rather, on ears which heard doctrines of only remote applicability. The membership figures of the NUWC, put at between 10,000 and 12,500 by the radicals and at 3,000 by the police, testify to that.[51] Sympathy was no substitute for consanguinity. There was a great chasm between the essentially *artisan* radicalism of Lovett, Watson and Hetherington, and the actuality of life in the dens of Limehouse and Shadwell which could not be filled. The first compromise came at the formation of the NUWC when the full title was agreed as the National Union of the Working Classes *and Others*. This fundamental betrayal came when the Farce Day was seen as a political demonstration. In the struggle against cholera, the poor were on their own.

9

Cholera and Society in Perspective

CHOLERA was to return in epidemic form three times after 1832; in 1848–9, 1853–4, and 1866. The second outbreak was to be far worse than the first. Although no completely reliable data are available, cholera killed at least 61,000 people in Britain in 1848–9, 53,000 in England and Wales, and 8,000 in Scotland. Total deaths in 1832 had numbered 31,000. Even taking population growth into account, the mortality rate from cholera in 1848–9 was higher than in 1832. The two following epidemics, however, were not as serious. In 1853–4, 26,000 deaths occurred, 10,000 of these in London. In 1866 there were 17,000 deaths, 6,000 in London.[1]

The curve of mortality from these four epidemics is strange; usually, when a virgin population is attacked, one would expect the highest mortality to occur in the first epidemic. But the second epidemic was at least twice as fatal as the first. One possible explanation for this was that a long period—sixteen years—elapsed between the epidemics. Amongst a population in which the age-structure was biased towards youth, a considerable proportion could not have had the opportunity of building up resistance to cholera before 1849. Britain thus was still virgin territory when cholera arrived a second time. But, with three epidemics between 1849 and 1866 which traversed the whole country, it seems possible that either the pool of potential victims began to diminish, or that some accommodation between organism and host began to occur.[2]

Another possibility was that cholera did not blanket the country so effectively in 1832 as it did in 1849. Omitting Scotland from what follows because of the absence of data, 293 towns and villages reported cases of cholera to the Central Board of Health in 1832; in 1848–9, about 750 places did so.[3]

Thirty-six English counties were infected in 1832, in which excluding London, about 16,000 people died. In 1848–9 and 1853–4, forty-two counties were infected, the mortality being, respectively, 40,000 and 10,000. Forty-one counties, the exception being Rutland, were infected in 1866, and, again, about 10,000 died.

The six counties unaffected in 1832 were all primarily agricultural (rural Surrey, Sussex, Hertfordshire, Northamptonshire, Herefordshire and Rutland). All were to be infected in 1848–9, although Hertfordshire had only seven deaths, and Rutland and Herefordshire one each. An outbreak in Hastings raised the number of deaths in Sussex, while 70 per cent of Northamptonshire deaths occurred in the towns of Northampton and Peterborough.[4] The total number of deaths in these six counties in 1849 came to 1,074, insufficient to explain the increased mortality of the epidemic on its own.

However, within certain counties which were only slightly infected in 1832, there was a significant increase in the number of deaths in 1849. The southern counties especially were attacked more severely. The five-fold increase in Kent occurred primarily in the Medway towns and in the southern coastal towns of Margate and Ramsgate. Further along the seaboard, Hastings, Portsmouth and Southampton raised mortality in Sussex and Hampshire. Taken together, the three counties suffered 226 deaths in 1832, and 1,809 in 1848–9.

Other regions to suffer much more severely in 1849 were the counties surrounding London (Essex, Middlesex, Surrey and Herfordshire), Somerset, Wiltshire, Cheshire and Monmouthshire. These eight counties suffered 382 deaths in 1832, and 4,235 in the second epidemic. Except for the last two mentioned counties, and Northampton, Herefordshire and Rutland, all the counties which suffered marginally or not at all in 1832, and relatively severely in 1849, were in the South, stretching from Somerset in the west to Essex in the east. This broad southern region's mortality in 1849 at least partly helps to explain the increased mortality in that year, for deaths rose from 482 in 1832, to 5,606 in the second epidemic. It accounts, therefore, for about 20 per cent of the additional deaths in the second epidemic in England and Wales.

A considerable proportion of the remaining excess of deaths

occurred in particular industrial regions. South Wales, especially the iron town of Merthyr, had more than 3,000 additional deaths in 1849, about 12 per cent of the excess. Fatalities in the West Riding also trebled, with Leeds and neighbouring Hunslet particularly badly hit. Sheffield was almost a success story, but fast-growing Bradford's mortality increased fourteen-fold over 1832, when only 30 died. Approximately 11 per cent of excess mortality in 1849 could be attributed to the West Riding.

But it was Lancashire which endured the greatest increase in cholera mortality, from nearly 3,000 deaths in 1832 to more than 8,000 in 1849, accounting for 21 per cent of the excess. Those textile towns which escaped unscathed in 1832 were visited by cholera in 1849, but only a handful of deaths resulted. Again, the water supply coming from the Pennines was their saviour. Manchester had only a hundred more deaths, but Wigan suffered very severely, and Liverpool was devastated. Having undergone a severe epidemic of typhus in 1847 in the wake of massive Irish immigration, Liverpool had more than 5,000 deaths from cholera in 1849, 3,800 more than in 1832. Liverpool alone accounted for about 15 per cent of excess provincial mortality in 1849.

The geographical picture of the second epidemic can be summed up as follows. Virtually every county in England was struck by cholera. There was a significant increase in mortality in the southern counties and those surrounding London. Some of the worst hit regions in 1832, such as Northumberland and Staffordshire, had increased deaths, but probably did not keep up with population rise. The mortality rates of most major towns were either similar to 1832, or slightly lower, except that Liverpool, Leeds and some towns which had grown enormously in the 1830s and 1840s, had greatly increased mortality. As in 1832, many smaller communities were infected, but it is not known if their mortality rates were higher than the bigger towns. Given the same conditions as prevailed in 1832, there is no reason to suppose that they fared any better. However, while these virgin townships and villages may have contributed as much as 40 per cent to the additional mortality in 1849, it was the large towns, such as Liverpool and Merthyr, with their grotesque and possibly atypical socio-economic conditions, on which cholera mostly thrived.

The 1854 epidemic was much more centralised, even though nearly every county was infected at some point. Deaths in the West Riding dropped dramatically, and mortality in the southern counties declined towards the 1832 level. Most of the larger towns had fewer deaths, but Liverpool, Merthyr and the Tyne region (where the water supply was far more polluted than in 1849)[5] fulfilled the conditions for cholera's rapid and deadly diffusion. In 1866, most counties had only a smattering of deaths, although Devon and Lancashire had significant mortality, while South Wales, especially Swansea and Neath, were particularly badly hit. Staffordshire, the scene of great outbreaks in 1832 and 1849, had only thirty deaths in 1866, on a par with the rural counties. Thus, on its final visit to Britain, cholera was a major problem only for London, Liverpool and South Wales.

However, even as late as 1866 cholera managed to infect nearly every county in England. Its means of diffusion, especially around the coast by ship, were still effective, but obviously cholera's 'ideal' conditions for spread within a community had begun to disappear soon after the second outbreak. It is hard not to conclude that, even allowing for possible changes in personal susceptibility and in the relationship between organism and host, the relatively simple preventive measures, such as settling reservoirs and filtered water, were beginning to be applied on a significant scale.

This brings us to a consideration of the influence of the sanitary reform movement on cholera's demise. There is no need here to tell the story of sanitary reform from the 1840s, as it has been recounted excellently by Finer, Lewis and Lambert, but it is necessary to consider the role of cholera in the movement's genesis and subsequent development. Many textbooks and monographs have stated that cholera acted as a catalyst for public health measures, and there is some truth in this, but only for the second epidemic, not the first.

As shown above,[6] central policy towards public health at the grassroots was circumspect in 1832. Encouragement was given and pressure placed on the local authorities, but only in the sphere of finance did the Privy Council act with prescription; usually most recommendations emanating from London remained permissive. Where cholera was taken seriously in the provinces, Orders in Council were usually strictly interpreted, but many local authorities did very little to prepare against the disease, and the tiny flower of voluntary enthusiasm, which bloomed towards the end of 1831, was crushed by the dead weight of local inertia.

It was an awareness of the strong feeling for local autonomy which prompted the permissive character of government policy in 1832, and there is little evidence to suggest that this was not the best approach. There was, for example, no movement at the end of the epidemic to continue the local boards of health, as the way which surplus money was used demonstrates. In Manchester, the Committee of the Cholera Relief Fund introduced a follow-up system whereby families of cholera victims were visited and relieved. As a result, a Provident Society was formed.[7] In St George Hanover Square, the £1,100 remaining from subscriptions were invested in government stock, and in 1833 was used to finance three soup kitchens.[8] In neither place, both of which were well organised in 1832, was there any suggestion that more than a continuation of traditional philanthropic action was necessary (and Manchester, also, had been the subject of James Kay's pamphlets).

If we except from the discussion for a moment particular individuals such as Kay in Manchester and Robert Baker in Leeds, on both of whom cholera had a galvanising effect, the 1832 epidemic failed miserably to generate amongst the middle-classes a recognition that public health reform was necessary. After 1832 they seemed to have forgotten everything and learned nothing. James Smith of Deanston, writing of Thomas Laycock's 1845 report on York for the Health of Towns Association, recognised this. The report showed, he wrote,

> a view of the generally careless and inefficient workings of the public authorities during a long period of time, and [demonstrated] that on several occasions, when disease became excessive, and the men in power and the better classes in general became alarmed for their own safety, they gave some attention to the undrained and filthy conditions of the localities and the abodes of the lower classes, and made some temporary efforts to remove the evils; but that no sooner had the impressive period of danger passed over them than the drainage and cleansing were neglected as before; that not only

> were the old places left in their former condition, but even where new dwellings were from time to time constructed, no measures appear to have been taken to erect them on higher and drier sites, or to prevent the recurrence of former evils by systematic draining and cleansing.[9]

What was lacking was a widespread understanding of the relationship between disease and social conditions. If a lesson was drawn from the epidemic it was that there was a need, not for sanitary reform, but for a reform in morals. Such an attitude, however, missed the essential point, which James Kay at least appreciated.

> Cholera can only be eradicated by raising the physical and moral condition of the community, in such a degree as to remove the predisposition to its reception and propagation, which is created by poverty and immorality. Were this notion, as it ought to be, widely diffused; did it become, as it will, the conviction of every intelligent man, what additional force would be added to the arguments suggested by sympathy and selfishness.[10]

But most of the educated classes were not to be convinced. It required an effort of will which many would not make, or at least would only do so either when the disease was imminent or when it was raging. Even after the second epidemic this attitude persisted. Thomas Frost, who witnessed the first two cholera epidemics, believed that a sense of fatalism, the old hand of God idea reinforced by Malthusian theory, had much to do with middle-class apathy. Writing after cholera had disappeared from Britain of the contaminated water supplies and impure atmosphere which had abounded, he said,

> But then we had been used to these evils since the days of the Plantagenets, and though they had become intensified with the increase of population and the growth of the large towns, had not Malthus taught us that epidemics of disease were one of the means used by divine providence to prevent the numbers of the human race exceeding the means of subsistence?[11]

Nor did the central government consider the possibility of a long-term policy towards public health after 1832. A final report, based on information from the few local boards which bothered to reply to a circular, was drawn up by the Central Board, but it was mildly self-congratulatory and made no reference to the need for a permanent central health authority. Sir David Berry used the same data in a paper given before the London Statistical Society, which was subsequently published posthumously in the first volume of the society's *Journal*, but again, no health policy was envisaged.[12] The relief felt because cholera had been successfully combated with temporary machinery, combined with the absence of a strong and well-coordinated provincial public opinion in favour of sanitary reform, ensured that the first cholera epidemic had few long-term repercussions. Why establish national public health machinery permanently when *ad hoc* measures had been comparatively successful in reducing the impact of cholera?

When cholera reappeared in the autumn of 1848, a very different administrative machinery existed to cope with it. In August 1848 the Public Health Act had been passed and in September the Nuisances Removal Act, which had clauses dealing with the presence of epidemic disease, had received the royal assent. The Public Health Act was the culmination of ten years work by Edwin Chadwick in the field of sanitary reform. The General Board of Health, which was established under the Act and consisted of Chadwick, Southwood Smith and Lords Ashley and Morpeth, had less success in combating cholera than its predecessor of 1832. This was partly because it depended on the local boards of guardians acting as temporary boards of health in the provinces. Unlike the voluntary boards of 1832, which consisted of interested members of the community who were frequently motivated both by humanitarian feelings and civic pride, and took their responsibilties towards the poor seriously in times of crisis, the Boards of Guardians had been established to protect the interests of the propertied against what they felt to be unreasonably high poor rates. They were unsuited to the role of custodians of the public health, which in practice meant the expenditure of rates. With little power to enforce its recommendations, the General Board of Health was forced to watch cholera march unopposed throughout the country in 1849.[13]

Nor did the General Board receive the same assistance from the medical community as its predecessor had in 1832. The

Central Board of Health, following Henry Halford's dismissal in November 1831, had pursued a policy which, while antagonising some medical practitioners who held extreme views of disease causation (contagionists and noncontagionists alike), had straddled the middle ground and thereby reduced the prospects of confrontation. It had, moreover, in Russell and Barry two respected and cholera-experienced physicians. In contrast, the General Board of Health had only one medical man in 1849 (Southwood Smith), who was an extremist in his views, although he had treated cholera patients in 1832. Chadwick, too, accepted Smith's simplistic view of disease causation and had made it the main plank of sanitary reform ideology in the 1840s. With the establishment of the General Board in 1848, the sanitary view of disease and the 'filth' theory of disease causation became 'official doctrine', but it was not a doctrine which was acceptable to a very significant portion of the medical profession. This is a point not sufficiently emphasised by historians, who have usually seen medical opposition to Edwin Chadwick as stemming from his lack of faith in medical science and the medical community. But it is clear from the medical journals of the time, especially the *Medical Gazette*, that while Chadwick's contempt for doctors was significant, there was still a strong body of opinion existing in medical circles which saw cholera as a contagious disease and was therefore critical of the premises underlying General Board planning. The Royal College of Physicians in Edinburgh, hostile to the pretensions of the General Board, believed that some of the most experienced practitioners in Scotland rejected the filth theory, and even Thomas Laycock of York, a strong supporter of the Health of Towns Association, was himself a contagionist when it came to cholera, and claimed that every cholera-experienced practitioner he had spoken to was of his persuasion.[14]

When the South London Medical Society debated the contagiousness of cholera in August 1849, 'a few hands were held up on either side, but the greater proportion of the members abstained from so expressing their opinions on the subject'. It was also admitted at the Royal Medical and Chirurgical Society that the contagiousness of cholera was still the *vexata questio* amongst the medical community.[15]

Medical practitioners were, then, both frustrated and somewhat demoralised in 1849, which did not help the General Board in implementing its policies. The medical officers of the Poor Law Unions, who bore the brunt of the epidemic in most towns, were specially embittered by their experiences. Dependent on the Guardians for their positions, they found that the Nuisances Removal Act, under which they operated against cholera, was sufficiently vague to allow the Guardians to refuse extra payment for their increased workload. Nor could the General Board persuade the Guardians to employ temporary assistants for the overworked medical officers.[16]

This is not to suggest that the medical community failed to live up to the high standards of their predecessors; rather, faced with a larger number of cases than in 1832, they became more aware of their relative impotence. Having a General Board at the helm which not only had little real weight but also espoused doctrines unamenable to many doctors, it is not surprising that some disillusionment occurred. Treatment remained much the same as in 1832, except that venesection was not practised; O'Shaughnessy's experiments were repeated with the same results, and the saline treatment in practice was found to be temporarily effective, although most patients still died.[17]

The measures undertaken against cholera in 1849 were, therefore, mainly unsuccessful, although such procedures in some towns as moving potential victims away from infected houses, a practice used in Edinburgh in 1832, may well have diminished mortality somewhat.[18] Chadwick's policy of flushing sewers repeatedly, as mentioned earlier, was enormously destructive and the encouragement of all suffering from premonitory diarrhoea to visit a doctor immediately, the basic recommendation of the Board of Health, probably had little effect.

However, although *The Times* complained in 1852 that 'the cholera was departed out of sight and mind and we have relapsed into indifference or something beyond',[19] the 1849 epidemic probably did encourage the inhabitants of many towns to apply to the General Board of Health to implement the Public Health Act in their region. The first effects were to be seen in the next epidemic, when mortality declined below the 1832 level. While, therefore, the emergency measures taken to combat cholera were not very effective, the prior existence of public health machinery enabled those who were jolted by the severity of the epidemic to pursue their demands for sanitary reform after 1849. Although the Public Health Act was unpopular for its centralising tendencies, concerned groups were better placed because of it to reform the basic sanitary conditions of their towns than their counterparts had been in 1832. But the process whereby this situation arose was influenced but little by cholera epidemics; the 1849 outbreak did not so much generate sanitary reform, so much as confirm the need for public health measures. What was possible under the Act was limited, but fortunately cholera was a disease which could be eradicated almost entirely by effective sanitary measures alone.

Given the vastly increased mortality from cholera in 1849, it would be expected that social attitudes towards the disease would have reflected greater concern and panic than in 1832. And, indeed, there is evidence that many of the responses of the first epidemic were repeated. The same general fears engendered in 1832 were repeated in 1848–49. Alarm and exaggerated rumours were again reported from Leeds and Bristol and in Salisbury 'the alarm was at its highest on Tuesday evening, owing to a great number of timid persons having been present from the country, who unwisely exaggerated the current reports and enhanced the public alarm. A case too, having occurred in the public market was the fruitful cause of much uneasiness.'[20] The residents of Clifton near Bristol were sufficiently concerned again to flee the city. In Mevagissey a Plymouth surgeon found that

> fear of the scourge had scarcely left a person in the town willing to assist those who were ill or to bury those who were dead. A scene of greater consternation could scarcely be witnessed. Many had fled from the spot to the neighbouring villages, while others had taken to the boats. . . . Many of the shops were closed, and persons who had been in the habit of attending the market with produce, refused to attend—looking on the village as a doomed spot.[21]

Those who had sailed to Fowey found they were refused permission to land and had to lie in their boats in great distress.

Family and friendship ties again came under stress. The Reverend Edward Jackson recounted the case of a Leeds man drunk from brandy staggering into his wife's death-chamber. The brandy had been the medicine for his wife given to him by the surgeon at the local workhouse.[22] In the South-West, reports were received of the dying being robbed of their blankets, while the attending surgeons had their pockets picked.[23] In Bere Alston, Devon, the local miners, having initially demanded the right of carrying their deceased friends to the graveside, became so panic-stricken at the intensity of the epidemic that no one could be found to put the coffins in the cart or to lead the horse.[24]

Many of the factors which stimulated the profusion of rumours in 1832 still existed in 1848–9. Admittedly Chadwick's General Board of Health tried to allay fears of contagion by a massive propaganda campaign defending the miasmatist position and by displaying hostility to the foundation of temporary isolation hospitals. Unconvinced, many towns established hospitals in 1849, which could have served as potential flashpoints for disturbances as in the first epidemic.[25] House-to-house visitation was never put into practice until the disease was at or past its height, and even the General Board had to admit that from a preventive viewpoint, the system was a failure.[26] Thus the use of middle-class visitors to working-class areas as a means of displaying class collaboration and of reducing tension was not possible in 1849. The necessity of the swift removal of the dead was also insisted on, although in Irish areas (as in the appositely-named Hairbrain Court in Whitechapel) wakes still continued.[27] Even a cynical attitude towards the medical profession still prevailed in some areas, as in Hull where the old rumour that doctors were paid more for treating patients who died than those who recovered again circulated.[28]

Yet, for all these similarities with the first epidemic, there was one essential difference in 1849; while there was fear and panic, there was no unrest in the country, which *The Times* had certainly expected.

> In our age the vast increase of population, the more than proportionate increase of luxury and wealth—the great contrast of conditions and fortunes—have all raised up elements of discord, contention and bitter strife . . . which, in a widespread pestilence, might now ferment into anarchy and ruin. The metropolis could not have suffered alone. It would have infected all England. We have escaped these evils. We have escaped anarchy. We have escaped national convulsion.[29]

In 1849 the country also escaped riots stimulated by cholera. This can be explained by reference to the decline of social tension, particular and local, which had generated disturbances in 1832. Of crucial importance was the changed relationship of the medical profession to the poor. Between 1832 and 1848 there had been a breakdown in the riot syndrome: anti-doctor feeling; fear; rumours; precipitating incident; action. All sections of the syndrome were present in 1849 but the core, the social tension, had diminished. Its decline should be seen in terms of the solution to the problem of finding bodies for dissection.

Warburton's Anatomy Bill became law in June 1832. Its purpose was to ensure that bodysnatching and burking died out and that a sufficient number of bodies were supplied to the schools of anatomy. Overseeing the Act's administration were two inspectors, Dr Craigie in Edinburgh and Dr James Craig Somerville in London. (With the former's dismissal for misconduct in 1836, Somerville became responsible for the whole country.)[30] For the ten years of Somerville's inspectorate (1832–42), the Act failed to work satisfactorily. It is true that no further cases of burking ever came to light, but reports of resurrectionists at work throughout Britain remained common until 1841.[31] These were not on the same scale as in the 1820s; nevertheless, they were significant, for their reporting prevented Somerville from achieving his aim of keeping the working of the Act a secret.[32] The Anatomy Act was permissive; bodies were handed over to the anatomy schools only with the agreement of the local parish officers. Moreover paupers, by signing a declaration, were free to opt out of the Act's provisions.

Somerville therefore aimed to allay prejudice, but his task was rendered immeasurably more difficult by the limited nature of the Act and the consequent selfish attitude of the anatomy surgeons. No procedures had been laid down for the distribution of the bodies which became available. Somerville's preference for distribution in accordance with numbers of students at each anatomy school was frequently upset by some teachers' penchant for adding the names of mythical students to their registers.[33] Moreover, many others deliberately short-circuited the system by making their own personal arrangements with the local parish officers, receiving unclaimed dead from the workhouse in return for free treatment for paupers. Unseemly squabbles amongst surgeons at vestry meetings in London resulted in the rapid decline of bodies available to the anatomy schools.[34] In the provinces, where the number of available bodies was always smaller and more of the dead were claimed by next of kin, the struggle for bodies was acute and resurrectionism remained necessary.[35]

The implementation of the Poor Law Amendment Act further increased Somerville's difficulties in London. In the popular mind both Acts were seen as part of an onslaught against the poor by a middle-class seeking social and cultural hegemony. It is at this stage, in the mid-1830s and in certain areas where the needs of local medical schools required the implementation of the Anatomy Act, that the whole question of the relationship between the poor and the medical profession develops temporarily from a diffuse and general suspicion of doctors towards an articulated manifestation of *class* consciousness. That this was only a transient phenomenon is perhaps explained, ironically, in terms of the opposition which the Anatomy Act provoked amongst segments of the local ruling class. The passing of the Poor Law Act, for example, engendered such antagonisms amongst the poor that many vestries refused to execute the provisions of the Anatomy Act, lest disturbances resulted. Moreover, the most effective attack on the Act came from a small group of dissidents within the medical teaching profession, whose activities had the side-effect of demonstrating that not all the middle-classes approved of this legislation.

At the centre of this agitation in London was the obscure figure of William Roberts. Roberts, who was probably the William Henry Roberts of 30, Upper Montagu Street elected as a select vestryman in St Marylebone in 1823,[36] first came to prominence in 1832 by claiming to have discovered a method of preventing the rapid decomposition of corpses. Although many authorities, including Somerville, were initially impressed with the technique, experiments proved it a failure and the government rejected Roberts' demand for £5,000 in return for forgoing his patent rights.[37] Roberts (wrongly) blamed Somerville for his failure and henceforth worked to blacken the inspector's name in the London vestries by publicly denouncing the Anatomy Act. According to Somerville, Roberts tried 'to blow up the anatomical schools, by placarding their nefarious activities', especially the disgusting mode of 'treating the remains and the mockery of the interment'.[38] Roberts held open meetings in a public house in Tottenham Court Road and personally visited workhouses to inform the poor of their right to opt out of the provisions in the Anatomy Act.[39]

Roberts was helped in his campaign by George Dermott, lecturer in anatomy in Charlotte Street, Soho, who had a personal grudge against Somerville, and by Thomas Tatum and John F. Foster of the Kinnerton Street school of anatomy.[40] They probably became involved with Roberts in order to attack a local rival school of anatomy run by Samuel Lane (both schools were negotiating to merge with St George's hospital).[41] Between 1839 and 1842 Roberts received information from Kinnerton Street which seriously damaged the working of the Anatomy Act in the Unions, especially in Marylebone where Foster was on the board of guardians and in opposition to the ruling party of radical petty tradesmen who saw the implementation of the Anatomy Act as a means of reducing the poor rate (every body used at an anatomy theatre was eventually buried at the teacher's and not the Union's expense).[42] Roberts' exposure of the surgeons' unfeeling and illegal methods of disposing of dissected bodies (Somerville admitted that Roberts' accusations were based on 'pretty correct information'),[43] resulted in the decline in the numbers of bodies obtained under the Act. Between 1832–3 and 1841–2 the supply from the London parishes fell from 394 to 216 and Somerville's alternative sources —hospitals, hulks, prisons, asylums and dwelling houses—could not make up the difference. Total supplies had been 609 in 1832–3; Somerville received 378 in his last year as inspector.[44] Somerville was right to claim that the Act had become 'a stalking horse for popularity and influence in the parishes, or the means of bigotry in some parochial or party squabble in the vestry'.[45]

Outside London, where rivalries between local teaching surgeons were not so bitter, the need for bodysnatchers, and their occasional exposure, kept the Anatomy Act in the public eye and resulted in more attacks on anatomy schools. In December 1833 a crowd attacked the Cambridge University anatomy theatre after the spreading of a rumour that a body had been obtained illegally. In fact the body had come from the local workhouse but the parish officers, frightened by the popular clamour, denied this. Professor Clarke and his colleagues, including the Vice-Chancellor, were forced to defend their premises against the crowd before magistrates arrived to read the Riot Act.[46]

In 1834 Somerville arrived in Hull to discover whether the local anatomy teachers had been dealing with a band of recently convicted resurrectionists. He found the walls of the anatomy theatre covered with 'many opprobrious epithets, designating the teachers as Burkers and their School a Burking shop'.[47] Although the teachers indignantly denied any connection with the bodysnatchers, the local authorities' refusal to implement the Anatomy Act had forced the surgeons to revert to obtaining bodies illegally. They nevertheless argued that agitation had been stirred up by 'the ignorance and prejudice of the lowest orders aided by certain malicious individuals'.[48] In the following year the Sheffield anatomy theatre in Eyre Street was completely destroyed by a crowd and the surgeons were forced, after ten years' work, to give up their private venture.[49]

Disturbances, of a less serious nature, were reported until 1841, by which time it was obvious that Somerville had failed in his purpose of keeping the running of the Act secret. The final straw was Roberts' demand for an enquiry into the corrupt appropriation of money by Somerville (the inspector was acquitted but the charges rankled), followed by his petition to Parliament in July 1842 complaining of the Act's failure. Hardly surprisingly, Somerville was dismissed soon afterwards. His successors, although possibly less successful than Somerville in obtaining bodies,[50] were able to implement the Anatomy Act in secrecy, for by the mid-1840s the struggles between the anatomy teachers had ended with the amalgamation of some of the private schools with local hospitals and with the demise of others. By the time the second cholera pandemic appeared on the horizon in 1847 there was no agitation which could stir the fears of the poor. When cholera struck in 1848–9 it engendered responses similar to those in 1832, except that riots and disturbances, generated by anti-doctor hostility, did not occur. The essential stability of British society in 1832 was confirmed in 1849.

Appendix

THE CHOLERA

Modern medical research has distinguished three forms of classic Asiatic cholera: choleraeic diarrhoea; cholerine; and the typical syndrome of classic cholera. All are caused by the entry into the intestine of the vibrio *V. cholerae*. The drinking of water contaminated with the excreta of cholera victims or the eating of food after contact with such victims are major channels of cholera's transmission and inadequate personal cleanliness an important contributory factor. Flies also act as carriers of the disease. Of the three types of cholera, choleraeic diarrhoea and cholerine are only mild forms of the disease. Both are present during a cholera epidemic, the former causing mere diarrhoea, although a victim's stools could contain an enormous number of cholera vibrios, while the latter shows all the premonitory symptoms of true cholera but omits some of the later stages. Neither is as fatal as true cholera.

True cholera progresses through three stages, the first being that of evacuation when there is a sudden onset of violent purging and vomiting of 'rice-watery' evacuations. In the second stage, that of collapse, there is acute dehydration, a profound collapse and the almost complete cessation of urine secretion. At the same time there is circulatory failure, a characteristic change in the patient's features (normally the skin becomes 'corrugated' and displays a bluish tinge), together with very painful muscular cramps. In the third stage, of reaction, there is either a rapid return to health, an imperfect reaction leading to death, or an excessive reaction leading to hyperpyrexia or uraemia and, usually, death.

Like all other bacterial infections, cholera's virulence is influenced by the physical and human environments in which it exists. Its endemic locations are Bengal, its original home, in the deltaic region of the Ganges and the Brahmaputra; the delta in Orissa State and Madras State; the Irrawaddy delta in Burma; and the Yangtse river in China. Cholera is endemic in these regions partly because of the surface-water system and partly because each has a densely-packed population at or near the coast, living in areas hardly more than fifty feet above sea level. *V. cholerae* also requires certain favourable climatic conditions in order to survive for any length of time. A high temperature and a suitably high atmospheric humidity promote its epidemic spread. Cooler weather diminishes the attraction of cold food and drink and reduces the number of flies which could act as vectors. A drier atmosphere also tends to kill the cholera vibrio on vegetables. The normal climatic conditions prevailing in Bengal make it a natural endemic focal point for cholera, especially in December and January, and March and April; conditions suitable for cholera's rapid dissemination in Britain would occur most frequently in August and September.

The human environment also plays its part in spreading cholera. Its long-distance transmission depends on systems of human communications, trade routes, pilgrim trails and migration paths. There can be little doubt that cholera first broke out of the Indian subcontinent and became pandemic in 1817 because of India's growing trade linkages with the world economy: overland into Russia, and by sea to China and Japan. Once settled in a new country, cholera's progress depends on the socio-cultural environment in which the population lives. Poverty and malnutrition, overcrowded dwellings, inadequate and polluted water supplies, inefficient or non-existent refuse disposal programmes and the absence of comprehensive sewerage and drainage systems, all—in varying ways and to varying degrees—may promote the epidemic spread of *V. cholerae*. At the level of personal human relationships daily contacts with neighbours, regular visits to the homes of family and friends, the traditional and worthy desire to visit the sick and the dead, regular attendance at church, chapel or secular institution, can occasion the extension of a disease which relies to a considerable extent on healthy carriers.

However, the linkages between the organism and its potential victims are not as strong as might be expected. *V. cholerae* is unable to withstand high temperatures, even very weak solutions of acid (including gastric juices with hyperacidity), disinfectants and most organisms found in decayed and decomposing organic matter. Yet the vibrio can survive for up to fifteen days in faeces, seven in earth dust and on moistened coal, twenty-one on dry coal, and for three days on raw cotton and cloth. Although capable of surviving for only a short period in filtered water, the vibrio can live for several weeks in spring water, for up to twenty days in river water and is, moreover, remarkably tolerant of low temperatures, even below freezing point. As water is the prime medium for the transmission of cholera, its durability in that environment is of crucial importance. One leading epidemiologist has written,

> There is little room for doubt that, provided conditions for the subsistence of *Vibrio cholerae* do exist, the temperature of the water, which in turn depends on the prevailing season, is one of the main factors, perhaps the principal factor, determining the length of survival of the organisms.

And as the water becomes warmer, the vibrio begins to multiply more quickly.

Eating and drinking habits are also important for the transmission of cholera within a community. Water offers the greatest danger, unless it is boiled before consumption. Hot drinks, such as tea, coffee and cocoa, if contaminated after cooling, can harbour the vibrio for many days. Contrary to the opinions of many nineteenth-century temperance reformers, spirit and beer drinking do not necessarily increase personal susceptibility. *V. cholerae* survives in beer for three hours and in wine for only fifteen minutes; spirits can possibly kill it in the intestine.

Certain foodstuffs are a suitable substratum for the cholera organism, but it is not true that poorer quality foods are *necessarily* more dangerous. Cholera can thrive on meat and fish, and can live for a month on best butter but only for a day on the low-grade acid variety. The vibrio dies on cheese and potatoes after two days, on sugar after three and on rye bread after one. Green vegetables are particularly dangerous because of the likelihood of their being washed in contaminated water.

ABBREVIATIONS

BHM	Bulletin of the History of Medicine
DNB	Dictionary of National Biography
EcHR	Economic History Review
EMSJ	Edinburgh Medical and Surgical Journal
HJ	Historical Journal
JHM	Journal of the History of Medicine
JLSS	Journal of the London Statistical Society
JRSS	Journal of the Royal Statistical Society
JSH	Journal of Social History
LMG	London Medical Gazette
LMPJ	London Medical and Physical Journal
LMSJ	London Medical and Surgical Journal
MH	Medical History
PDSH	Plymouth, Devonport and Stonehouse Herald
PMG	Poor Man's Guardian
P&P	Past and Present
TPMSA	Transactions of the Provincial Medical and Surgical Association

Notes

Chapter 1
PREPARATIONS
(pp. 7–26)

1. Hobson, *World Health and History*, 76.
2. Corbyn, *Epidemic Cholera in India*, 4–5.
3. Pollitzer, *Cholera*, 17; Banerjea, 'Cholera in Uttar Pradesh.'
4. *The Lancet*, i, 1831–2, 242.
5. *Ibid.*, 243–9; Pollitzer, *Cholera*, 18–22.
6. Haytesbury to Aberdeen, 29 September 1830, PC 1/4395(1).
7. Haytesbury to Aberdeen, 7 October 1830, *ibid*; McGrew, *Russia and the Cholera*, 76–8.
8. Brockington, *Public Health in the Nineteenth Century*, 1.
9. McDonald, 'History of Quarantine', 22–44.
10. Haytesbury to Palmerston, 5 January 1831, PC1/4395(1); Pym to Greville, 26 January 1831, *ibid.*
11. Greville, *Memoirs*, ed. Reeves, Vol. 2, 154.
12. Greville to Halford, 16 June 1831, PC1/4395(1).
13. Winterbottom, 'Thoughts on Quarantine and Contagion', 63–4.
14. P.C. to Walker, 14 January 1831, PP, xvii, 1831. Greville thought Walker to be 'a very useless and inefficient agent'. *Memoirs*, 154.
15. Walker's reports were dated 4 and 17 March and were printed in PP, xvii, 1831.
16. Report of Dr Albers, March 1831, *ibid.*
17. Greville, *Memoirs*, 154; Winterbottom, 'Thoughts on Quarantine', 79.
18. Pym to Greville, 7 June 1831, PC1/4395(1).
19. Halford *et al* to Greville, 9 June 1831, *ibid.*
20. First Report of Royal College of Physicians, 15 June 1831, *ibid.*
21. Second Report of RCP, 18 June 1831, *ibid.*; P.C. to Russell, 17 June 1831, PC1/2660.
22. Brockington, *Public Health*, 2–13.
23. P.C. to Halford, 18 June 1831, PC1/4395(1). In the official

copies of communications there are only ten names, Pelham Warren's being omitted. But he was certainly on the Board from its inception.

24. For Halford, see *DNB*, vii, 923; Macmichael and Munk, *Gold Headed Cane*, 140–59.
25. *DNB*, xx, 875–6.
26. *Ibid.*, xii, 673–4; Clark, *History of RCP*, 655.
27. *Ibid.*, 633; *DNB*, xii, 60 and ix, 1038–9; Munk, *Roll of RCP*, Vol. 3, 144–9.
28. *DNB*, xvi, 527–8.
29. McGrigor, *Autobiography and Services; DNB*, xii, 546–9, iii, 414–15, xii, 1183–4; Clark, *History of RCP*, 663.
30. *The Lancet*, ii, 1830–1, 433–4.
31. Instructions to Board of Health, 21 June 1831, PC1/2660.
32. Greville, *Memoirs*, 160.
33. Minutes of Central Board of Health, 25 June, 4 July 1831; Hearncorn to H.O., 29 June 1831, HO44/24.
34. Minutes of Central Board of Health, 8 August, 19 September 1831; Lewis to P.C., 8 August 1831, PC1/4395(1).
35. Minutes of Central Board of Health, 24, 28 June 1831.
36. *Ibid.*, 23 June 1831. They received copies of the regulations drawn up when the plague (actually yellow fever) had invaded Malta in 1813 and Gibraltar in 1829.
37. Hobsbawm and Rudé, *Captain Swing*; Fraser, 'Agitation for Parliamentary Reform'; Jones, *Before Rebecca*; Williams, *The Merthyr Rising*.
38. Marshall to Board of Health, 23 July 1831, PC1/101. Marshall was a Port Glasgow surgeon, and cholera was thought to have arrived in the town from Riga in a flax consignment. Dr Robert Daun, an experienced army doctor, was sent there by the Privy Council, but found only cases of English cholera. Marshall rejected this diagnosis and published a justificatory pamphlet, which made him 'a standing joke in the north'. Minutes of Central Board, *passim*; Marshall to Halford, 23 July 1831, PC1/4395(1); Daun to P.C., 27 July 1831, *ibid., LMG*, 22 October 1831.
39. Greville, *Memoirs*, 160.
40. *The Lancet*, i, 1831–2, 125.
41. Russell and Barry to Central Board, 4 August 1831, PC1/101.
42. *Examiner*, 11 September 1831.
43. Chad to P.C., 18 September 1831, PC1/101; Greville, *Memoirs*, 197.
44. *Examiner*, 4, 18 September, 2 October 1831; *Annual Register*, 1831, 438–9.

45. *Examiner*, 30 October 1831; Minutes of Central Board, 21 October 1831; *The Times*, 24 October 1831.
46. *Ibid.*, 20 August 1831.
47. *LMG*, 29 October 1831.
48. *The Lancet*, i, 1831–2, 113.
49. Minutes of Central Board, 23 July, 4 and 8 August 1831, PC1/101; *LMG*, 22 October 1831.
50. Gaulter, *Cholera in Manchester*, 29. Information received from Jonnès in Paris showed that Hamett had deliberately falsified the number of deaths in Danzig. Jonnès to Pym, 1 December 1831, PC1/108.
51. Macmichael to Seymour, 6 October 1831, HO31/17.
52. *London Gazette*, 20 October 1831.
53. Preliminary Resolutions of Board, n.d. (but pre-October 20), HO31/17.
54. Pym to Jonnès, 14 November 1831, PC1/108.
55. Thompson, *Making of English Working Class*, 808.
56. Minutes of Central Board, 19 October 1831, HO31/17.
57. *PDSH*, 5 November 1831; *The Lancet*, ii, 1830–1, 820; *ibid.*, i, 1831–2, 156–7; *Examiner*, 6 November 1831.
58. *Quarterly Review*, November 1831, 265–73.
59. Bright to Central Board, n.d., PC1/101; Central Board to P.C., 27 June 1831, *ibid.*; *The Lancet*, ii, 1830–1, 476–7; Returns of Streets and Places in Metropolitan Police Districts, 22 July 1831, PC1/114.
60. *The Lancet*, i, 1831–2, 304.
61. *Ibid.*, 20.
62. *Ibid.*, ii, 1830–1, 433–4.
63. House of Commons Sessions Papers, Finance Accounts, 1831–2, 473.
64. List of Doctors and surgeons on furlough from India, PC1/4395(2).
65. *The Lancet*, i, 1831–2, 17.
66. Macmichael, *Is Cholera Spasmodica Contagious?*, 3.

Chapter 2
THE DIFFUSION OF CHOLERA THROUGH BRITAIN
(pp. 27–49)

1. The progress of the epidemic can be traced in the Public Record Office files PC1/105 and HO31/17.
2. Clanny, *Hyperanthraxis*, 4–5; Minutes of Central Board, 12, 13, 16 December 1831; Miller & Porbock to P.C., 1 December 1831, PC1/93.

3. Greenhow, *Cholera in Newcastle and Gateshead*, 90–2.
4. Minutes Metropolitan Sanitary Commission, 1847–8, 1; *The Lancet*, i, 1831–2, 706.
5. *Ibid.*, 739–43.
6. *Ibid.*, 740–1; Minutes of Central Board, 13 February 1832; Minutes of St Saviour Southwark Board of Health, 13 February 1832.
7. Minutes Metropolitan Sanitary Commission, 2.
8. Minutes of Central Board, 21 February, 18 March, 2 April 1832; S.C. on Metropolitan Sewers, 1834, 60–1; Minutes of City of London Board of Health, 2 March 1832; P.C. to Bethnal Green District Surgeons, 7 March 1832, PC1/94.
9. Minutes of Central Board, 21 April 1832.
10. There are three sets of data for this phase of the epidemic in London, in PC1/108, PC1/114, and daily records in PC1/105. I have used the last source here, as it appears to be the most comprehensive.
11. See the file of letters in PC1/95; *Morning Chronicle*, 2 to 26 July 1832; Report of City Board of Health, 3 August 1832, PC1/114.
12. Minutes of Central Board, *passim*; Cholera Returns of Great Britain, PC1/108; Hewitt, 'Cholera in Beith, 1833–4', 150.
13. Siegfried, *Germs and Ideas*, 16.
14. *Sheffield Iris*, 27 December 1831.
15. Riddell to Edinburgh Board of Health, 26 December 1831, PC1/107.
16. Minutes of Central Board, 12 January 1832.
17. Samuel, 'Comers and Goers', 123–50.
18. Minutes of Central Board, 5 April 1832.
19. *The Times*, 6 February 1832; *PDSH*, 4 February 1832.
20. Durey, *Cholera in York*, 10.
21. *Staffordshire Advertiser*, 13 June 1832.
22. Streeten, 'Report on Worcester in 1832', 390.
23. Gatherer, 'Socio-Medical Study of the First Cholera Epidemic in Britain', D.M. thesis, University of Aberdeen 1960, 158–9; *Staffordshire Advertiser*, 23 June 1832; *PDSH*, 21 July 1832.
24. Samuel, 'Comers and Goers', 136.
25. H.O. to Baillie, 29 August 1832, HO43/42; H.O. to Woodward, 30 August 1832, *ibid.*
26. Jones, 'Cholera in Wales', 284.
27. *Ibid.*, 283; Stokes, *Cholera in Sheffield*, 182.
28. *Leeds Mercury*, 9 June 1832; Jewitt, *History of Plymouth*, 406.
29. Radzinowicz, *History of English Criminal Law*, Vol. 4, 22–5.

30. *Cholera Gazette*, 14 January 1832.
31. Circular from Edinburgh Board of Health, n.d. (early 1832), PC1/103.
32. Minutes of Central Board 1 December 1831, 10 January, 28 February 1832; House of Commons Sessions Papers, Finance Accounts 1831–2, 479; Central Board to Davidson, 29 February 1832, PC1/94.
33. Anon, *Remote Cause of Cholera,* 55.
34. Christison, 'Arrangements of Edinburgh Board of Health', 1832.
35. *Medico-Chirurgical Review*, xvi, 1832, 572.
36. Gaulter, *Cholera in Manchester*, 5–6. But in February 1832 the Manchester Board of Health had contacted their counterparts in Preston, Huddersfield and Rochdale suggesting that they acted on the question of vagrants. Proceedings of Manchester Board of Health, 15 February 1832.
37. Minutes of Central Board, 11 April 1832; *Victoria County History of Staffordshire*, vii, 127; Hamilton-Jenkin, *Cornwall and Its People*, 341–2.
38. *PDSH*, 1 September 1831; Shapter, *Cholera in Exeter*, 250.
39. Select Vestry Minutes, Norton (Yorks), 15 June 1832.
40. See file of letters in PC1/94; Treasury to P.C., 12 April 1832, PC1/4395(3).
41. These figures do not include data from the collieries and villages around Newcastle, for which there is no separate information.
42. Robson, *Urban Growth*; Law, 'Growth of Urban Population in England and Wales, 1801–1911', 125–43.
43. Baker, *Leeds Board of Health*, 11–14; *Leeds Intelligencer*, 27 September 1832.
44. Shapter, *Cholera in Exeter*, 223.
45. Durey, *Cholera in York*, 8; *Staffordshire Advertiser*, 28 July 1832; Gaulter, *Cholera in Manchester*, 110; Ogier Ward, 'Cholera in Wolverhampton 1832', 370; Underwood, 'Cholera in Yorkshire 1832', 604.
46. *Liverpool Chronicle*, 23 June 1832.
47. Durey, *Cholera in York*, 13–14; Shapter, *Cholera in Exeter*, 75–7; Smith, *Report on York*, 17; Bonser, 'Spas, Wells and Springs of Leeds', 29–50.
48. *Leeds Mercury*, 21 July 1832; *Morning Chronicle*, 21 July 1832.
49 It is true, however, that some newspaper proprietors refused to publish news of cholera when local outbreaks first occurred. See below.

50. *Leeds Intelligencer*, 9 August 1832; *Leeds Mercury*, 28 July 1832; *Cobbett's Weekly Political Register*, 5 May 1832; Place Papers, BM Add Ms 27791, 379–80; Gaulter, *Cholera in Manchester*, 108.
51. Minutes of Central Board, 11 January 1832; Ward, *Factory System*, 159.
52. Chadwick, *Sanitary Condition of Labouring Population*, 293.
53. *Local Reports on Sanitary Condition 1842*, 264–5.
54. Chadwick, *Sanitary Condition*, 105–6, 363–4, 411; *Local Reports 1842*, 194.
55. *Ibid.*, 193.
56. Baines, *History, Directory of Lancaster*, Vol. 2, 534.
57. Second Report of Health of Towns Commission 1845, 112; Woodhead, *Huddersfield Water Supplies*, 46–54.
58. The pureness of the water supplies enabled millowners to claim that it was safer for the workforce to be in the mills than in their homes. Gaulter, *Cholera in Manchester*, 119–20.
59. *Local Reports, Scotland, 1842*, 87–8.
60. *Ibid.*, 216.
61. Snow, *On Cholera*, 117–18.
62. *Local Reports, Scotland, 1842*, 209.
63. Chadwick, *Sanitary Condition*, 135–42.
64. Snow, *On Cholera*, 117–18.
65. Riddell to P.C., 28 January 1832, PC1/105.
66. Smiles, *Samuel Smiles*, 30.
67. Rennie to P.C., 15 April 1832, PC1/107; Pyper to H.O., February 1832, HO44/49.
68. Data for Sunderland can be found in the Privy Council Papers, for Manchester in an appendix to Gaulter, and for York in Durey, *Cholera in York*.
69. *Liverpool Courier*, 15 August 1832; Stokes, *Cholera in Sheffield, passim.*

Chapter 3
CHOLERA AND THE ENVIRONMENT: THE CASE OF LONDON
(pp. 50–76)

1. Snow, *On Cholera*, 16–20.
2. Rosen, 'Disease, Debility and Death', 629.
3. Rosen, 'People, Disease and Emotion', 18.
4. Rosenberg, 'Cholera in Nineteenth-Century Europe', 454.
5. A. J. Taylor ed., *The Standard of Living in Britain in the Industrial Revolution.*

6. Chevalier, 'Le Choléra à Paris', in *Le Choléra*, 31–4; Zacke, *Kolera Epidemien*, 175.
7. S.C. Metropolitan Sewers 1834, iii, 23; Webbs, *Statutory Authorities*, 68–9, 86.
8. S.C Metropolitan Sewers 1834, 36–41.
9. *Ibid.*, 3, 13; T. Davis, *Sewage or Drainage, passim.*
10. S.C. Metropolitan Sewers 1834, 87; Webbs, *Statutory Authorities*, 100–1; Minutes of Surrey and Kent Commission of Sewers, 16 December 1831.
11. Minutes of Metropolitan Sanitary Commission, 1847–8, 13–19.
12. Report to Privy Council, February 1832, PC1/104.
13. Jephson, *Sanitary Evolution of London*, 17.
14. Report of Westminster Visiting Committee, 6 December 1831, HO44/24; Minutes of Westminster Commission of Sewers, 6 January 1832.
15. S.C. Metropolitan Sewers 1834, 128, 167.
16. Minutes of Metropolitan Sanitary Commission, 41.
17. Jephson, *Sanitary Evolution*, 18.
18. Minutes of Central Board, 16 November 1831; Register of the Court of Tower Hamlets Commissioners of Sewers, 2 December 1831, 24 February 1832; Hutchinson to P.C., 3 December 1831, PC1/103; S.C. Metropolitan Sewers 1834, 127, 162–4; *The Times*, 25 October 1831.
19. Hutchinson to P.C., 3 December 1831, PC1/103.
20. Jephson, *Sanitary Evolution*, 9.
21. City of London Board of Health Committee Papers, 13 January 1832; S.C. Metropolitan Sewers 1834, 33–4, 113–15.
22. Minutes of Holborn & Finsbury Commission of Sewers, 27 January 1832.
23. *Ibid.*; S.C. Metropolitan Sewers 1834, 19; Barton, *Lost Rivers of London*, 52, 110.
24. S.C. Metropolitan Sewers 1834, 149–50.
25. Minutes of Metropolitan Sanitary Commission, 18.
26. Minutes of Rolls Board of Health, 18 November 1831, 23 July 1832.
27. Minutes of St Mary Stratford Board of Health, 23 November 1831; Minutes of Tottenham Board of Health, 19 January 1832.
28. Minutes of St George Hanover Square Board of Health, 24 November 1831; Minutes of Rolls Board of Health, 18 November 1831; Report of Westminster Committee, 6 December 1831; Minutes of City Board of Health, 7 November 1831; Minutes of Metropolitan Sanitary Commission, 1.
29. S.C. on Supply of Water to the Metropolis 1828; Snow, *On Cholera*, 57–60.

30. S.C. on Metropolitan Water 1828, 13; Pollitzer, *Cholera*, 165.
31. *Ibid.*, 856.
32. Quoted in *ibid.*, 851.
33. Buer, *Health, Wealth and Population*, 101.
34. S.C. on Metropolitan Water 1828, 15–47; S.C. on Metropolitan Water Supplies, 1834, 64.
35. S.C. on Metropolitan Water 1828, 36; S.C. Metropolitan Sewers, 1834, 31; Oram, 'Old London Bridge', 551.
36. Jephson, *Sanitary Evolution*, 15.
37. *Ibid.*, 22.
38. *Ibid.*, 22–3; Minutes of Metropolitan Sanitary Commission, 13.
39. *The Unknown Mayhew*, edited Thompson & Yeo, 21.
40. Minutes of Metropolitan Sanitary Commission, 1–2. There was a large sewer outfall at this point.
41. There was possibly some under-registration of deaths in Christchurch.
42. Snow, *On Cholera*, 64.
43. Lampard, 'The Urbanising World', *Victorian City*, Vol. 1, 13.
44. Price-Williams, 'The Population of London, 1801–81', 398; Dyos, *Victorian Suburb*, 50.
45. George, *London Life in the Eighteenth Century*, 400.
46. Minutes of Metropolitan Sanitary Commission, 13; Minutes of Rolls Board of Health, 18 November 1831, 7, 15 August 1832.
47. Redford, *Labour Migration in England*, 120–1; Shannon, 'Migration and the Growth of London', 81.
48. George, *London Life*, 122–3; Redford, *Labour Migration*, 115; *The Times*, 3 March 1832; Minutes of St George H.S. Board of Health, 8 December 1831.
49. Hansard, 3rd series, x, 1832, 390; Vestry Minutes of St Matthew Bethnal Green, 4 November 1831; P.C. to Treasury, 15 March 1832, PC1/94.
50. Gough to P.C., 16 February 1832, PC1/4395(3).
51. North-East St Giles' District Visiting Society to Spring Rice, 3 March 1832, PC1/4395(3); Greville to Spring Rice, 7 March 1832, *ibid.*
52. *Morning Chronicle*, 21, 26 July 1832.
53. See below.
54. Vestry Minutes of St Paul Covent Garden, 23 February, 15, 26 March 1832.
55. Report of Westminster Committee, 6 December 1831.
56. Anderson to P.C., 23 March 1832, PC1/105.
57. *The Times*, 7 October 1848, quoted in Finer, *Chadwick*, 347.
58. Chadwick, *Sanitary Condition*, 120.
59. Finer, *Chadwick*, 347.

60. For the 1866 cholera epidemic in London see Report of Epidemic Cholera in England, 1866; Eyler, 'William Farr on the Cholera', 79–100; Luckin, 'The Final Catastrophe—Cholera in London, 1866', 32–42.
61. Walker, *Gatherings from Graveyards*; Chadwick, *Report on the Sanitary Condition of the Labouring Population of Great Britain: Supplementary Report on the Practice of Interment in Towns*, 1–23.
62. Chevalier, *Labouring Classes*, 203.
63. *Ibid.*, 152, 206, 228, 465; Chadwick *Sanitary Condition*, 149–50.

Chapter 4
THE MEDICAL POLICE AT WORK IN 1832
(pp. 77–100)

1. The other members were Edward Stewart, Sir William Pym and Lieutenant Colonel J. Marshall.
2. Minutes of Central Board, 31 October, 4 November 1831.
3. Greville to Local Boards, 11 November 1831, PC1/102.
4. Keith-Lucas, 'Some Influences Affecting the Development of Sanitary Legislation in England'; Hennock, 'Urban Sanitary Reform a Generation before Chadwick?'; Buer, *Health, Wealth*, 200, 206.
5. Hammonds, *Town Labourer*, 57.
6. Webbs, *Statutory Authorities*, 353.
7. Minutes of Central Board, 14 November 1831.
8. The Central Board nevertheless acted as if cholera's importation had been proved.
9. Fenwick to Power, 12 December 1831, House of Commons Sessions Papers 1831–2, 476; Lamb to P.C., 20 December 1831, *ibid.*; Riddell to P.C., 21 January 1832, PC1/103; Central Board to P.C., 27 January 1832, *ibid.*
10. Clissold to P.C., 26 September 1831, PC1/101; Mayor of Lynn to Melbourne, 1 November 1831, HO44/24; Boston Board of Health to P.C., 15 November 1831, PC1/105; Marston to P.C., 18 November 1831, BM Add Ms 27967; Carter to Melbourne, 1 November 1831, HO44/24; Coppard, *Cottage Scenes*, 4–6.
11. Minutes of City Board of Health, 11 November 1831; Minutes of City Medical Committee, 1831.
12. Minutes of Central Board, 12 January 1832; Riddell to Central Board, 21 January 1832, PC1/103.
13. Greville, *Memoirs*, 264.
14. Minutes of Central Board, 30 November, 13 December 1831, 11

February 1832; Galbraith to Tenby Board of Health, 2 April 1832, PC1/103.

15. *Yorkshire Gazette*, 3 December 1831.
16. Minutes of Rolls Board of Health, 4 November 1831; Langford, *Birmingham Life*, 495; Christison, 'Edinburgh Board of Health', cclv. The Central Board recommended that officially constituted boards should have between nine and fifteen members. Minutes of All Saints Poplar, 15 November 1831.
17. Minutes of Westminster Commission of Sewers, 2 December 1831; Minutes of Surrey and Kent Commission of Sewers, 16 December 1831.
18. Shapter, *Cholera in Exeter*, 85.
19. Christison, 'Edinburgh Board of Health', cclv–cclxi.
20. Minutes of Rolls Board of Health, 15 November 1831.
21. See especially Report of Subcommittee of Norwich Board of Health, 27 January 1832, BM Add Ms 27967.
22. For example, many of the district reports in Manchester were either imperfect or not compiled at all. Proceedings of Manchester Board of Health, 18 January 1832.
23. *London Gazette*, 14 November 1831.
24. Owen, *English Philanthropy*, 96; Poynter, *Society and Pauperism*, 3.
25. Barry to P.C., 28 November 1831, PC1/103; Vestry Minutes of St Matthew Bethnal Green, 16 November 1831. As a last act of charity before he died in January 1832, one man gave £10, a bullock and a cartload of turnips to the Lanark Board of Health. *LMSJ*, i, 1832, 64.
26. Briggs, 'The Language of Class', 44.
27. Minutes of Central Board, 22 and 26 November 1831.
28. Christison, 'Edinburgh Board of Health', cclxiii-cclxv; *Yorkshire Gazette*, 24 December 1831; Minutes of Portsoken Board of Health, 21 February 1832.
29. Kirkman Gray, *English Philanthropy*, 152.
30. Minutes of City Board of Health, 1 November 1831.
31. Christison, 'Edinburgh Board of Health', cclxiii; Vestry Minutes of Greenwich, 2 August 1832; Shapter, *Exeter*, 185–6; *Yorkshire Gazette*, 24 December 1831.
32. Christison, 'Edinburgh Board of Health', cclxxx.
33. *Yorkshire Gazette*, 24 December 1831; Minutes of St Mary Stratford Board of Health, 8 December 1831.
34. *Blackwood's Magazine*, xxvii, 1830, 92.
35. Christison, 'Edinburgh Board of Health', cclxxxviii.
36. Hansard, 3rd series, x, 1832, 337.
37. *Ibid.*, 268.

38. Minutes of Rolls Board of Health, 30 January 1832; Hewitt, 'Cholera at Beith', 148; Proceedings of Manchester Board of Health, 19 December 1831.
39. *Ibid.*, 8, 11 February, 23 August, 4 September 1832.
40. Minutes of City Board of Health, 29 February, 15 March 1832. By the end of March there were seven temporary hospitals in the city, five of which were controlled by ward boards of health, catering for 76 patients.
41. Evans to P.C., 30 March 1832, PC1/105; Minutes of Central Board, 11, 17, 30 April 1832.
42. *Ibid.*, 16 November 1831, 21 February, 3 April 1832.
43. Central Board to Carson, 15 May 1832, PC1/95; Central Board to Horace, 7 July 1832, *ibid.*
44. Minutes of Tardebigge Board of Health, 30 September 1832; Coppard, *Cottage Scenes*, 50.
45. *Ibid.*, 19–23.
46. Stokes, *Cholera in Sheffield*, 111.
47. York Corporation House Book, 1, 25 July 1832.
48. District Inspectors to Central Board, 9 January 1832, PC1/114; Superintendents of Police to P.C., January 1832, PC1/103.
49. Central Board to Greville, 23 January 1832, PC1/93.
50. Pearson to Lansdowne, 16 June 1832, PC1/114; Minutes of City Board of Health, 13 July 1832; Report from City Board of Health, 3 August 1832, PC1/114; Stern, 'Holloway Prison', *Studies in London History*, eds Hollaender & Kellaway, 447–50.
51. Central Board to Richards, 27 June 1832, PC1/95.
52. *The Lancet*, ii, 1831–2, 85; Stokes, *Sheffield*, 37; Proceedings of Manchester Board of Health, 20 June 1832; Streeten, 'Report on Worcester', 391; Ogier Ward, 'Cholera in Wolverhampton', 375.
53. The Manchester leypayers spent £50 cleaning the notorious Little Ireland in 1832, but Engels' description twelve years later shows that any improvement was purely transitory. Engels, *Condition of Working Class*, 60–1.
54. Proceedings of Manchester Board of Health, 31 October 1832.
55. Gutchen, 'Local Improvements and Centralisation', 86.
56. Bullen to Arthur, 2 March 1832, PC1/107; Campbell to Arthur, 4 March 1832, *ibid.*
57. Arthur to Central Board, 16 April 1832, *ibid.*; Minutes of Central Board, 23 February 1832.
58. Arthur to Central Board, 16 April 1832, PC1/107.
59. Greville to Central Board, 13 July 1832, PC1/95.
60. For squabbles on Gorbals Board of Health see *Glasgow Chronicle*, 19 March 1832; Lawrie to Central Board, 24 April

1832, PC1/105. Also, Morris to Central Board, 5 April 1832, *ibid*; Worcester Board of Health to Central Board, 12 April 1832, *ibid.*

61. Trench to Central Board, 28 March 1832, PC1/105; Hicks to Central Board, 10 April 1832, *ibid.*
62. Hansard, 3rd series, x, 1832, 338–46.
63. Greville to Ware, 28 February 1832, PC1/4395(3); Central Board to Treasury, 21 February 1832, PC1/94; Spring Rice to Greville, 10 March 1832, *ibid.*; Minutes of Central Board, 6 April 1832; Central Board to Brougham, 21 February 1832, PC1/93; Minutes of St Saviour Southwark Board of Health, 23 February, 19 April 1832; Greville to Treasury, 18 February 1832, PC1/93; Fox Maule to Spring Rice, 7 April 1832, PC1/4395(3).

Chapter 5
CHOLERA, MEDICINE AND THE MEDICAL COMMUNITY
(pp. 101–134)

1. Shyrock, *Development of Modern Medicine*, 24; Ackerknecht, 'Anti-contagionism', 565.
2. Waddington, 'General Practitioners and Consultants in Early Nineteenth-Century England', *Health Care and Popular Medicine,* eds Woodward & Richards, 165–6.
3. S.C. on Medical Education 1834, 35 (evidence of Macmichael).
4. Holloway, 'The Apothecaries Act, 1815: A Reinterpretation', *Medical History*, x, 1966.
5. Inkster, 'Marginal Men: Aspects of the Social Role of the Medical Community in Sheffield, 1790–1850', *Health Care*, 128.
6. Sprigge, *Thomas Wakley*; Brook, *Battling Surgeon.*
7. For a fuller discussion of the Anatomy Act see Durey, 'Bodysnatchers and Benthamites', 200–25.
8. Woodward, *To Do the Sick No Harm*; Sigsworth, 'Gateways to Death?', *Science & Society, 1600–1900*, ed. Mathias.
9. *The Lancet*, ii, 1831–2, 88.
10. Winslow, *Conquest of Epidemic Disease*, 173–4.
11. Ackerknecht, *Short History*, 222; Winslow, *Conquest*, 203.
12. *EMSJ*, xvi, 1820, 109; McDonald, 'Quarantine', 25.
13. Macnamara, *Asiatic Cholera*, 4.
14. *EMSJ*, xvi, 1820, 111–12.
15. McDonald, 'Quarantine', 27.
16. *Examiner*, 1 March 1832.
17. Ackerknecht, 'Anticontagionism', 574.
18. Barry, 'Remarks on the Gibraltar Epidemic', *London Medical*

and Physical Journal, x, 1831, 475–94, xi, 1831, 1–23.

19. Langdon-Brown, *Some Chapters in Cambridge Medical History*, Cambridge 1946, 77; Greenwood, 'Miasma and Contagion', *Science, Medicine and History: Essays... in Honour of Charles Singer*, ed. Underwood, Vol. 2, London 1953, 502.
20. *The Lancet*, i, 1831–2, 261.
21. Macleod, editor of the *London Medical Gazette*, was known to the *Lancet*'s readers as 'The Yellow Goth', and Wakley called the *Gazette* 'the Weekly Excrescence'. Eckman, 'Anglo-American hostility and American medical literature of the nineteenth century', 38–9.
22. Barry, *Experimental Researchers*; Munk, *Roll*, iii, 214–6; *EMSJ*, xxvii, 1827, 214.
23. *EMSJ*, xvi, 1820, 460–2; Macmichael, *Cholera Contagious?*, 27–8; Chambers, 'Three lectures on cholera, delivered to the students of St George's Hospital, February 1832', *LMG*, vii, 1849, 325–6.
24. Kennedy, *History of Contagious Cholera*; Orton, *An Essay on the Epidemic Cholera of India*, 314. The first edition had been published in Madras in 1820.
25. *LMG*, 5 November 1831. See also *The Lancet*, i, 1831–2, 173; Anon, *Remote Causes of Cholera*, 1-2.
26. Kuhn, *Structure of Scientific Revolutions*, 15.
27. Rosen, 'Disease and social criticism; a contribution to a theory of medical history', 7.
28. *The Lancet*, ii, 1831–2, 153.
29. *Ibid.*, 84; Alderson, *Cholera at Hull*, 2.
30. *LMG*, 12 November 1831; *The Lancet*, i, 1831–2, 303; *LMSJ*, vii, 1831, 483.
31. Macmichael, *Cholera Contagious?*, 13. See also *The Lancet*, i, 1831–2, 300; *ibid.*, ii, 1830–1, 769–70.
32. Barry, 'Remarks on Gibraltar Epidemic', 478–9.
33. *LMSJ*, vii, 1831, 483–4.
34. *DNB*, x, 904–5; *The Lancet*, ii, 1830–1, 422; Pettigrew, *Biographical Memoirs*, Vol. 2, 8.
35. *Medico-Chirurgical Review*, xvi, 1832 268, 274, 484; *LMSJ*, vii, 1831, 481; *The Lancet*, i, 1831–2, 339.
36. *Medico-Chirurgical Review*, xvi, 1832, 267.
37. *LMG*, 14 January 1832.
38. Corbyn, *Cholera in India*, 5; Boyle, *Treatise on Cholera*, 27–8; *EMSJ*, xv, 1819, 360–1. Tytler returned to England in 1833 with his original ideas unchanged. See *The Lancet*, i, 1833–4, 57–72.

39. *EMSJ*, xxxviii, 1831, 188–9.
40. Gaulter, *Cholera in Manchester*, 133.
41. Rosen, 'Disease, Debility and Death', 635.
42. Proceedings of the Central Board of Health, 18 December 1832, PC1/2662.
43. *The Lancet*, ii, 1831–2, 149–50; *Medico-Chirurgical Review*, xvi, 1832, 556.
44. Winslow, *Conquest*, 182.
45. For water as a medium see Anon, *Remote Causes*, 25–6; Report of Bristol Board of Health, 24 January 1833, PRO PC1/102. The carrier concept was first suggested in India. Corbyn, *Cholera in India*, 83.
46. *LMG*, 19 November 1831.
47. *Ibid.* See also Kendrick, *Cursory Remarks on the Present Epidemick*, 12.
48. Rosenberg, *The Cholera Years: The United States in 1832, 1849, and 1866*, 75, n.2. See also Rosenberg, 'The Cause of Cholera: aspects of etiological thought in nineteenth-century America', 337.
49. *The Lancet*, ii, 1830–1, 820.
50. *LMSJ*, viii, 1832, 14.
51. *EMSJ*, xv, 1819, 365–6; King, 'The Blood-letting Controversy: a study of the scientific method', 4–5; Howard-Jones, 'Cholera Therapy in the Nineteenth Century', 374–7.
52. Niebyl, 'The English Bloodletting Revolution, or Modern Medicine Before 1850', 464–83.
53. Howard-Jones, 'Cholera Therapy', 374.
54. For help with the following I am very grateful to Laurence Hall, M.D., B.S., M.R.A.C.P., D.T.M. & H., M.R.C.P., of Mersey General Hospital, Tasmania. He is not responsible for any of the interpretations placed on his advice in this chapter.
55. Niebyl, 'English Bloodletting Revolution', 479. I could find little evidence in the journals to suggest that bleeding to excess was a common phenomenon.
56. Bloodletting was shown to be safe, wrote Benjamin Walsh in 1819, 'by the strongest of all arguments—ocular demonstrations of its safety'. Quoted by Niebyl, 'English Bloodletting Revolution', 472.
57. Howard-Jones, 'Cholera Therapy', 380–1.
58. *The Lancet*, i, 1831–2, 18.
59. Goodman & Gilman, *The Pharmacological Basis of Therapeutics*, 3rd ed., 1016. See also Langtry, 'The 1832 Epidemic of Asiatic Cholera in New Haven Connecticut', 475.
60. Langtry, 'Cholera in New Haven', 475.

61. Alderson, *Cholera at Hull*, 2.
62. Armstrong and Edgar, *Observations on Malignant Cholera*, 18–26; Mackenrot to H.O., 4 March 1832, HO44/25; *Medico-Chirurgical Review*, xvi, 1832, 276; *The Lancet*, i, 1832/33, 44; *EMSJ*, xv, 1819, 361–2.
63. The data can be found in Durey, 'A Social History of the First Cholera Epidemic in Britain, 1831–3', University of York D.Phil., 1975, 377.
64. Benenson, 'Cholera', 113.
65. Lambert, *Simon*, 245.
66. O'Shaughnessy, 'Blue Epidemic Cholera', 369.
67. Lewis to Maclean, 18 May 1832, PC1/103.
68. *The Lancet*, ii, 1831–2, 594–5; Anderson to Barry, 21 June 1832, PC1/103.
69. Coppard, *Cottage Scenes, passim.*
70. *Ibid.*
71. Blackman, 'Popular Theories of Generation: the evolution of "Aristotle's Works". The study of an anachronism', *Health Care*, 56–88.
72. Niebyl, 'English bloodletting', 469–70.
73. Stevens, 'On the Efficiency of Saline Agents in the Treatment of West Indian Fevers', *The Lancet*, i, 1831–2, 553.
74. *Ibid.*, ii, 1831–2, 455–7.
75. *Ibid.*, i, 1831–2, 592.
76. Lewis to Maclean, 18 May 1832; Lewis to Central Board, 23 May 1832, PC1/103.
77. The argument in Manchester was between Dr James Kay (later Kay-Shuttleworth) and Dr Henry Gaulter, both of whom published works on cholera in 1832. Their clash concerned the use of cholera data collected by the Manchester Board of Health (Kay was a contagionist, Gaulter a strong noncontagionist). Proceedings of Manchester Board of Health, 28 March 1832. For Liverpool, see *Liverpool Courier*, 7, 14, 28 March 1832.
78. *Hull Portfolio*, 12 June 1832.
79. *The Lancet*, i, 1831–2, 18.
80. Howard-Jones, 'Cholera Therapy', 380.
81. Alderson, *Cholera at Hull*, 2.
82. Howard-Jones, 'Cholera Therapy', *passim.*
83. The only exceptions to this opinion consist of two surgeons, one from Manchester and one from Liverpool, who resigned from their respective Boards of Health, because they feared they would lose their regular custom if it were known they were treating cholera cases.
84. See for example *The Times*, 6 February 1832; Minutes of St

George Hanover Sq. Board of Health, 23 July 1832. Many surgeons in the smaller communities were, no doubt, paid by the parish to visit the surrounding hamlets daily. For one example, see Minutes of Huntington Parish (Yorkshire), 15 July 1832.

85. Howard-Jones, 'Cholera Therapy', 386; McKeown, 'A Sociological Approach to the History of Medicine, 342.
86. The only known occasion when a surgeon experimented on his patients was in Wakefield, when the parish surgeon justified his actions by claiming that as his patients were paupers, they were suitable guinea pigs. Sharman to Central Board, PC1/102. Sir David Barry commented on the margin of this letter, 'Highly improper' and 'Not fit for publication'.
87. In some areas medals were struck for practitioners as a mark of respect for their actions in 1832. By contrast, in Beith during the epidemic of 1834, the Beith Humane Committee denounced the local doctors whose patients were 'drugged with infernal opium pills, laudanum injections and drenched with drops of brandy', and called in the quack doctor Knox Stewart. Nevertheless, of the 205 cases, 105 still died. Hewitt, 'Cholera in Beith', 150.

Chapter 6
CHOLERA AND THE PROPERTIED CLASSES
(pp. 135–154)

1. Greville, *Memoirs*, 154–6; Keer-Brown to Melbourne, 24 June 1831, HO44/24.
2. *The Times*, 18 June 1831.
3. Quoted in Inglis, *Poverty and the Industrial Revolution*, 268.
4. *The Times*, 27 June 1831.
5. *The Lancet*, ii, 1830–1, 421–2.
6. Greville, *Memoirs*, 160.
7. In terms of modern psychology, choleraphobia would represent reactions to the first (warning) phase before a possible disaster. Apprehension occurs when conditions arise from which personal danger may result. Stress leads either to repression of anxiety or to patent over-reactivity (denial or terror). Choleraphobia was symptomatic of the latter reaction and occurred amongst those suffering from a 'precarious general emotional situation'. Chapman, 'Introduction to Contemporary Disaster Research', *Man and Society in Disaster*, eds Baker and Chapman, 7–10.
8. Allport and Postman, *Psychology of Rumour*, 159.
9. *Ibid.*, 34; Kerckoff, 'Theory of Hysterical Contagion', *Human*

Nature and Collective Behaviour, ed. Shibutani, 83; Lefebvre, *The Great Fear of 1789*, 60.

10. *The Times*, 29 October 1831; *PDSH*, 5, 12 November 1831; *Sheffield Independent*, 12 November 1831; Gloucester Board of Health to Central Board, 26 November 1831, PC1/105; Gibson to Barry, 31 December 1831, PC1/103; Grosse, *A Surgeon in the Early Nineteenth Century*, 137.
11. *The Times*, 14 November 1831.
12. *PDSH*, 17 December 1831; *The Lancet*, i, 1831–2, 124.
13. *Morning Chronicle*, 17 February 1832; *The Times*, 16 February 1832.
14. *Sheffield Independent*, 12 November 1831.
15. *The Lancet*, i, 1831–2, 672.
16. *The Times*, 31 January 1832.
17. *Newcastle Chronicle*, 3 December 1831; Renny to Arthur, 26 March 1832, PC1/107.
18. Minutes of Central Board 22 and 24 December 1831, 28 January 1832; Alderson, *Cholera at Hull*, 6–9.
19. Lawrie, *Cholera in India, Sunderland, Newcastle and Gateshead*, 22.
20. Modern psychologists would claim that only one overt response was possible: 'separation from the threatening aspects of the feared object, accomplished by flight from the object, at one extreme, and conquest, at the other'. Sarnoff & Zimbardo, 'Anxiety, Fear and Social Affiliation', *Current Studies in Social Psychology*, ed. Steiner and Fishbein, 478.
21. Edith, Marchioness of Londonderry, *Frances Anne*, 173–4.
22. Baehrel, 'Épidémie et Terreur: histoire et sociologie', 354.
23. *Examiner*, 19 February 1832; Greville, *Memoirs*, 267.
24. Printed Minutes of City of London Common Council, 3 August 1832; *Morning Chronicle*, 11, 24 July 1832; *PMG*, 14 July 1832; *Leeds Intelligencer*, 5 July 1832.
25. *Leeds Mercury*, 21 July 1832.
26. Greville, *Memoirs*, 316.
27. *PDSH*, 14 July 1832; *The Cornubian*, 21 August 1832.
28. Rev. W. Leigh, quoted in Underwood, 'History of Cholera in Britain', 166–7; *Leeds Mercury*, 1 September 1832.
29. *Yorkshire Gazette*, 21 July 1831; *Morning Chronicle*, 11 July 1832.
30. *PDSH*, 2 June 1832; Latimer, *Annals of Bristol*, 187; Coppard, *Cottage Scenes*, 112.
31. For the Bath mob, led by the Amazonian Carroty Kate, see Singer, *Seventy Years a Showman*, 45–52.
32. *Leeds Mercury*, 11 August 1832.

33. Clanny, *Hyperanthraxis*, 13; *LMG*, 4 February 1832.
34. Kell, *Cholera at Sunderland*, 21–3.
35. *Ibid.*, 24; Kell to McGrigor, 2 and 3 September 1831, PC1/4395(1).
36. Kell, *Sunderland*, 27–9; Kell to McGrigor, 9 November 1831, PC1/4395(2).
37. Clanny, *Hyperanthraxis*, 13–20; Kell, *Sunderland*, 30–3; Kell to McGrigor, 26 and 27 October 1831, PC1/4395(2); *The Times*, 5 November 1831.
38. Clanny, *Hyperanthraxis*, 42; Kell, *Sunderland*, 36; Minutes of Central Board, 3 November 1831.
39. Kell, *Sunderland*, 39–40; Daun to P.C., 8, 9 November 1831, HO31/17.
40. Copy in City of London Board of Health Committee Papers. See also *Newcastle Courant*, 12, 19 November 1831; *Sunderland Herald*, 12 November 1831; *The Times*, 7 November 1831.
41. J. Stevenson to A. Stevenson, 9 November 1831, City Board of Health Committee Papers.
42. *Sunderland Herald*, 12 November 1831.
43. Kell, *Sunderland*, 49.
44. Daun to P.C., 11 November 1831, PC1/4395(1).
45. Resolutions of Merchants and Shipowners, 11 November 1831, PC1/4395(2); Daun to P.C., 15 November 1831, PC1/103.
46. *EMSJ*, xxxviii, 1832, 89–90.
47. Williamson to Melbourne, 14 November 1831, PC1/103.
48. Londonderry to Pym, 27 November 1831, *ibid.*
49. Minutes of Central Board, 17 and 21 November, 27 December 1831, 5 January 1832.
50. Barry to P.C., 28 November 1831, PC1/103.
51. Barry to Pym, 28 November 1831, *ibid.*
52. Evans to Peek Bros, n.d., City Board of Health Committee Papers.
53. Minutes of Central Board, 29 November, 5 December 1831; *Newcastle Chronicle*, 3 December 1831.
54. At the unconscious rather than the socio-cultural level, denial of cholera can be seen as a clear example of repression, which occurs 'when an idea or experience is forgotten, excluded from consciousness, or relegated to the realm of the unconscious'. Lifton, 'The Sense of Immortality', *Explorations in Psychohistory*, eds. Lifton and Olson, 153.
55. Proceedings of Manchester Board of Health, 21 December 1831.
56. Vestry Minutes, Christchurch Surrey, 22 March, 5 April 1832.
57. Vestry Minutes, St Clement Danes, 7 March 1832.

58. Vestry Minutes, St Paul Covent Garden, 23 February 1832. The placard was reprinted in *Cobbett's Weekly Political Register* and *The Examiner.* For the text, see below.
59. Vestry Minutes, St Paul Covent Garden, 23 February 1832.
60. Baehrel, 'La Haine de Classe', 354.
61. See also Ogier Ward, 'Cholera in Wolverhampton', 375, where the iron foundries were closed down.
62. *The Times*, 3 March 1832. In Haddington, Lady Elcho 'actually ordered the gates to be shut to prevent any intercourse with the inhabitants . . .'. McDonald to Stewart, 30 December 1831, PC1/107.
63. *The Times*, 5 March 1832.
64. *Wolverhampton Chronicle*, 22 August 1832.
65. Allison to Central Board, 21 November 1832, PC1/103.
66. *Idea of the City in Nineteenth-Century Britain*, ed. Coleman, 58–61; Carnall, *Southey and His Age*, 184–5.
67. Quoted in Morris, 'Organisation and Aims of the Principal Secular Voluntary Organisations of the Leeds Middle Class, 1830–51', Oxford D.Phil. 1871, 105–6.
68. *York Herald*, 9 June 1832.
69. *Yorkshire Gazette*, 21 July 1832.
70. *Ibid.*, 14 July 1832.
71. Coppard, *Cottage Scenes*, 25, 56.
72. Kitson Clark, *Churchmen and the Condition of England*, 74.
73. Jones, 'Cholera in Wales', 283–6.
74. Kendall, *Origins of the Primitive Methodist Church*, 106.
75. Thompson, *Cholera is Contagious*, 7.
76. Stephens, *Life and Letters of Dean Hook;* Stranks, *Dean Hook; Sketches of the Life of Edward Jackson of Leeds*, ed. Sykes.
77. Coppard, *Cottage Scenes*, 35–6; *Stafford County Herald*, 27 August 1832.
78. *Bristol Mercury*, 4 August 1832.
79. *Wolverhampton Chronicle*, 12 September 1832.
80. *The Examiner*, 7 January 1832.

Chapter 7
THE PEOPLE AND THE CHOLERA: (i) THE PEOPLE, AUTHORITY AND THE MEDICAL PROFESSION
(pp. 155–184)

1. Baehrel, 'Épidémie et Terreur', 113–14.
2. *Ibid.*, 121.
3. Chevalier, *Labouring Classes*, 22.
4. Chevalier, 'Le Choléra à Paris', 12–13.

5. Ackerknecht, 'Anticontagionism', 566; Niebyl, 'English Blood-letting', 469; Rosenberg, 'Etiological Thought', 335.
6. *The Times*, 20 February 1832; Baker, *Leeds Board of Health*, 9; Gregory to P.C., 19 February 1832, HO31/17; Bagnell to H.O., 22 July 1832, HO44/25.
7. Gaulter, *Cholera in Manchester*, 136.
8. *The Times*, 6 January 1832.
9. Gaulter, *Manchester*, 55. Mrs Bostock and her family were then taken to the reception house. When they all died within a few days, the neighbours' anger was turned on the doctors. Proceedings of Manchester Board of Health, 12 June 1832.
10. Girdlestone, *Seven Sermons*, xii.
11. Gaulter, *Manchester*, 86–7.
12. *The Times*, 1 February 1832; Minutes of Metropolitan Sanitary Commission, 14, 25; Shapter, *Cholera in Exeter*, 245–6.
13. Lizars, *Cholera Asphyxia*, 57–8.
14. Burne to Arthur, 1 March 1832, PC1/107.
15. *True Sun*, 2 June 1832; *The Lancet*, ii, 1831–2, 270.
16. *Liverpool Chronicle*, 2 June 1832; *Yorkshire Gazette*, 9 June 1831; *True Sun*, 2 June 1832.
17. *Liverpool Courier*, 6 June 1832.
18. *Ibid.*
19. Baehrel, 'La Haine de Classe', 355.
20. Shapter, *Cholera in Exeter*, 237.
21. It is noteworthy that when it came to finding buildings for use as cholera hospitals and owners of suitable property complained, the Central Board always replied that they had no intention of interfering with private property rights.
22. Clanny, *Hyperanthraxis*, 50; Scarborough Board of Health to Central Board, 28 December 1831, PC1/105; Longmate, *King Cholera*, 38.
23. *Cobbett's Weekly Political Register*, 17 March 1832.
24. See, e.g., Stedman Jones, 'Working-Class Culture and Working-Class Politics', 473.
25. Malinowski, *Magic, Science and Religion*, 52–3; Lifton, *Death in Life*, 493. See also Lewis, *Death in the Sanchez Family*, 36. 'Flies were beginning to gather over the body and I brushed them away. I couldn't bear the scene any longer. Everything oozed of death. I went outside.'
26. Malinowski, *Magic*, 52–3; Lifton, *Death*, 493.
27. Henderson, *Folk Lore of the Northern Counties*, 40; Hole, *English Folklore*, 51.
28. *Morning Chronicle*, 15 February 1832; Henderson, *Folk Lore*, 36–7.

29. Malinowski, *Magic*, 53.
30. Smart to H.O., 24 November 1831, HO44/49; *Wolverhampton Chronicle*, 8 August 1832.
31. Hole, *Folklore*, 50.
32. *Liverpool Chronicle*, 16 June 1832; *Liverpool Courier*, 13 June 1832; Pearson to Lansdowne, 16 July 1832, City Board of Health Letter Book, 89–92.
33. *Examiner*, 19 February 1832; Hill, *Seventy Two Years in Tottenham*, 6; City Board of Health Minutes, 8 August 1832.
34. Greville to Branston, 27 March 1831, PC1/94.
35. City Board of Health Committee Papers, 21 July 1832; Peek to City Board of Health, *ibid.*
36. *PDSH*, 18 February 1832
37. *Republican and Radical Reformer*, 15 September 1832.
38. Stokes, *Cholera in Sheffield*, 31–2; City Board of Health Minutes, 23 July 1832.
39. Pearson to Bishop of London, 16 July 1832, City Board of Health Letter Book.
40. *Examiner*, 11 and 18 March 1832; Stokes, *Sheffield*, 31; *Morning Chronicle*, 18 February 1832; *Yorkshire Gazette*, 28 July 1832.
41. Hole, *Folklore*, 54–5; Shapter, *Cholera in Exeter*, 249; Salmon to Arthur, 22 February 1832, PC1/107.
42. City Board of Health Committee Papers, 18 July 1832; *York Herald*, 14 July 1832; Shapter, *Exeter*, 236, 249; Branch Johnson, *Prison Hulks*, 134.
43. Mant, 'Medical Definition of Death', *Man's Concern with Death*, ed. Toynbee, 17, 19, 24.
44. *The Times*, 11 February 1832.
45. *Examiner*, 26 August, 2 September 1832.
46. Evans to Peek Bros, 3 January 1832, City Board of Health Committee Papers.
47. *Ibid.* See also *Leeds Mercury*, 6 October 1832; Bullen to Central Board, 17 January 1832; Arthur to Central Board, 2 March 1832, PC1/105.
48. *Newcastle Chronicle*, 19 November 1831; Shapter, *Exeter*, 247.
49. *Cholera Gazette*, 14 January 1832; Mant, 'Medical Definition of Death', 17.
50. Quoted in *ibid.*, 15.
51. Greville, *Memoirs*, 222; Daun to P.C., 29 January 1832, PC1/103; Daun to P.C., 23 November 1831, HO44/29; Clanny, *Hyperanthraxis*, 42–4.
52. Caton to Barry, 8 January 1832, PC1/103.

53. *Hull Portfolio*, 26 May 1832; Renny to Arthur, 14 March 1832, PC1/107; *Yorkshire Gazette*, 9 and 16 June 1832; *Leeds Mercury*, 6 October 1832; *PDSH*, 21 and 28 July 1832; *Staffordshire Advertiser*, 11 August 1832.
54. Durey, 'Bodysnatchers and Benthamites', 200–25.
55. S.C. on Anatomy 1828, 85. There were also 900 students in Edinburgh, 300 in Glasgow, 80 in Manchester, 40 in Liverpool and Birmingham, and about 20 in Bristol and Exeter.
56. *Ibid.*, 71.
57. Quoted in *Diary of a Resurrectionist*, ed. Bailey, 132.
58. Cole, *Things for the Surgeon*, 4, 15–16.
59. Bailey, *Diary*, 148–9.
60. S.C. on Anatomy 1828, 17–18.
61. Cole, *Things*, 30–4, 161–2.
62. S.C. on Anatomy 1828, 17.
63. *The Times*, 10 January 1829, 9 April, 19 June 1830, 2 April 1831; S.C. on Anatomy 1828, 30, 40.
64. Badham, *Christian Beliefs about Life and Death*, 47–8.
65. For a fictional account of an Irish wake, where the body was not buried until a missing leg was found, see Cordell, *The Fire People*, 11–13.
66. S.C. on Anatomy 1828, 72.
67. *The Times*, 26 December 1831; *Yorkshire Gazette*, 31 December 1831; Mitchell, 'Anatomical and Resurrectionist Activities in North Scotland, 417–29.
68. Cole, *Things*, 23.
69. S.C. on Anatomy 1828, 147–50.
70. *The Times*, 1, 8 January, 2, 12 and 13 February 1829; *Annual Register*, 1829, 20; Cole, *Things*, 117–23.
71. *The Times*, 20 January, 2 February 1829; Altick, *Victorian Studies in Scarlet*, 114.
72. *The Times*, 6, 7 December 1831; Frost, 'Burkers and Body-snatchers', *The Doctor in History*, 170–8.
73. The desperation of the snatchers to obtain bodies was shown by the fact that although supplies dropped, seven different gangs of resurrectionists were arrested in London and its vicinity between January 1830 and March 1831. *The Times, passim.*
74. *Examiner*, 26 February, 11 and 18 March, 1 April 1832; *Morning Chronicle*, 5 July 1832; Houlton to Melbourne, 30 March 1832, HO61/6; Greville, *Memoirs*, 285.
75. *Liverpool Chronicle*, 2 June 1832; *Liverpool Courier*, 6 June 1832; *Yorkshire Gazette*, 9 June, 25 August 1832; *True Sun*, 2 June 1832; *Bristol Mercury*, 11 August 1832; *Bristol Mirror*, 11 August 1832; *Sheffield Mercury*, 29 July 1832; Stokes,

Sheffield, 23–4, 34, 152; Gaulter, *Cholera in Manchester*, 38–9.

76. *Annual Register*, 1832, 44–5; *Leeds Intelligencer*, 29 March 1832; *Liverpool Courier*, 4 April 1832; *North Briton*, 31 March 1832; *Cobbett's Weekly Political Register*, 7 April 1832; Arthur to McKinley, 5 April 1832, PC1/107.
77. Proceedings of Manchester Board of Health, 19 July 1832.
78. *Cosmopolite*, 8 September 1832; *PMG*, 8 September 1832; *True Sun*, 6 September 1832; *Liverpool Chronicle*, 12 September 1832; *Liverpool Courier*, 12 September 1832; H.O. to Turner, 8 September 1832, HO43/42; Jordan, *Life of Joseph Jordan*, 133.
79. Thompson, 'Moral Economy of the Crowd', 78.
80. Place Papers, BM Add MS 27828, fos. 263, 284. Place also noted at the time of the trial of Bishop and Williams that the people had a bitter hatred of all 'in any way connected in anatomical studies'.
81. *The Times*, 22 December 1831.
82. Bailey, *Diary*, 69.
83. *The Times*, 19 April 1832.
84. *Liverpool Courier*, 4 April 1832; Peacock, 'York and the Resurrection Men, 4–5; Larks, *Plymouth Medical Society*, unpaginated.
85. *The Times*, 15 April, 26 December 1831; *Yorkshire Gazette*, 31 December 1831; H.O. to Sheffield Anatomy Lecturers, 17 February 1835, HO83/1.
86. Allison to Central Board, 21 November 1832, PC1/103.
87. Baehrel, 'La Haine de Classe', 358.
88. McGrew, *Russia and the Cholera*, 110, 117.
89. *Annual Register*, 1831, 438–9; *Gentleman's Magazine*, September 1831, 263.
90. *Bristol Mercury*, 11 August 1832; Latimer, *Annals of Bristol*, 186–7.
91. Turner, *The Inhumanists*, 52.

Chapter 8
THE PEOPLE AND THE CHOLERA: (ii) THE CHOLERA IN SOCIAL AND POLITICAL CONTEXT
(pp. 185–200)

1. Eversley, 'Le Choléra en Angleterre', 157.
2. Cholera Returns of Great Britain, PC1/108.
3. *Wolverhampton Chronicle*, 15 August, 12 September 1832; Longmate, *King Cholera*, 113; Hamburger, *James Mill*, 184–5; *PMG*, 15 September 1832.

4. Foster, *Class Struggle*, 99; Prothero, 'William Benbow and the Concept of the "General Strike" ', 150.
5. Rowe, 'Class and Political Radicalism in London, 1831–2', 34. The middle-class radicals included both Classical Economists and Utilitarians who 'at least until the 1830s . . . were united in both an ideological and a personal sense'. Taylor, *Laissez-faire and State Intervention in Nineteenth-Century Britain*, 34.
6. Rowe, 'Francis Place and the Historian', 47–9.
7. Hamburger, *James Mill*, 51. Cf. Thomas, 'James Mill's Politics: the "Essay on Government" and the Movement for Reform', 249–50.
8. Wallas, *The Life of Francis Place*, 287.
9. Greville, *Memoirs*, 217–18.
10. *Ibid.*, 286.
11. *The Examiner*, 13 November 1831; *The Lancet*, i, 1831–2, 377–8.
12. *The Examiner*, 13, 20 November 1831.
13. *Ibid.*, 13 November 1831.
14. *Ibid.*, 20 November, 11, 18 December 1831, 8 April 1832; Finer, *Chadwick*, 34; Finer, 'The transmission of Benthamite ideas, 1820–50', *Studies in the Growth of Nineteenth-Century Government*, ed. Sutherland, 15.
15. *The Examiner*, 18 December 1831, 11 March 1832.
16. Finer, *Chadwick*, 20; *The Autobiography of Francis Place*, ed. Thale, 283–5.
17. *The Times*, 16 February 1832.
18. *The Examiner*, 8 January 1832, 20 November 1831.
19. Weiner, *The War of the Unstamped*, 147; Prothero, 'Benbow', 151–2; Tholfsen, *Working Class Radicalism in Mid-Victorian England.*
20. Thompson, *Making*, 816; *The Times*, 16 October 1831; Hamburger, *James Mill*, 85.
21. Prothero, 'Benbow', 147–8.
22. Place Papers, BM Add. MS 27791, fo.25, quoted in Rowe, 'Francis Place', 58–9.
23. Thompson, *Making*, 768.
24. *Cosmopolite*, 14 July 1832.
25. *Cobbett's Weekly Political Register*, 25 February 1832.
26. *The Examiner*, 20 November 1831.
27. *Cobbett's Weekly Political Register*, 25 February 1832.
28. *PMG*, 25 February 1832; *Poor Man's Advocate*, 14 July 1832.
29. *PMG*, 18 February 1832.
30. *The Lancet*, i, 1831–2, 706.
31. *PMG*, 7 January 1832.

32. Weiner, *War of the Unstamped*, 144.
33. *Republican and Radical Reformer*, 15 September 1832.
34. *PMG*, 18 February 1832.
35. Lovett, *Life and Struggles of William Lovett*, 62.
36. Wearmouth, *Some Working Class Movements of the Nineteenth Century*, 62.
37. *Morning Chronicle*, 5 November 1831.
38. *PMG*, 11 February 1832.
39. Place Papers, BM Add. MS 27791, fo.377.
40. *Republican*, II, vii, May 1832.
41. *True Sun*, 16 March 1832; Lovett, *Life*, 64. No weapons, colours or ribbons were permitted.
42. Place Papers, BM Add MS 27791, fo.379.
43. *PMG*, 18 February 1832.
44. *Ibid.*, 24 March 1832; Lovett, *Life*, 64.
45. *Morning Chronicle*, 22 March 1832.
46. *PMG*, 24 March 1832; Place Papers, BM Add. MS 27791, fos.383–6.
47. *Ibid.*, fos.388–9.
48. *True Sun*, 22 March 1832.
49. *PMG*, 24 March 1832.
50. *Ibid.*
51. Hamburger, *James Mill*, 250.

Chapter 9
CHOLERA AND SOCIETY IN PERSPECTIVE
(pp. 201–215)

1. Longmate, *King Cholera*, 180, 195, 222.
2. See e.g. McNeill, *Plagues and Peoples, passim.*
3. Report of General Board of Health on Epidemic Cholera, 1850, 151–6.
4. Creighton, *History of Epidemics*, Vol. 2.
5. Snow, *On Cholera*, 106–7.
6. See above.
7. Report of Committee of Manchester Cholera Relief Fund, 11 April 1833.
8. Minutes of St George Hanover Sq. Board of Health, 4 January 1833.
9. Smith, *Report on York*, 2.
10. Kay, *Moral and Physical Condition of Working Classes in Manchester*, 12.
11. Frost, 'Reminiscences of the cholera', *The Doctor in History*, ed. Andrews, 189–90.
12. Barry, 'On the Statistics of Cholera', *passim.*

13. Report of General Board of Health, 1850, 79–84.
14. *LMG*, ix, 397.
15. *Ibid.*, 433; viii, 1849, 510.
16. *Ibid.*, 21–4.
17. *Ibid.*, 513.
18. Report of General Board of Health, 1850, 124–5.
19. Lambert, *Simon*, 184.
20. *The Times*, 20 July 1849. Between eight and ten thousand also fled Hull. Snow, *On Cholera*, 101.
21. *PDSH*, 28 July 1849.
22. *Life of Edward Jackson*, ed. Sykes, 56; Frost, 'Reminiscences of Cholera', 184.
23. *PDSH*, 21 July 1849.
24. *Ibid.*, 8 September 1849.
25. Report of General Board of Health, 1850, 129–32; *PDSH*, 4 August 1849.
26. Report of General Board of Health, 1850, 109–10.
27. *Ibid.*, 43; Minutes of General Board of Health, 19 January 1849.
28. Longmate, *King Cholera*, 164–5.
29. *The Times*, 27 September 1849; Report of General Board of Health, 1850, 124.
30. Durey, 'Bodysnatchers and Benthamites', *passim.*
31. Inspector of Anatomy's Letter Books, *passim*; *The Times*, 11 March 1836; Fourth Annual Report of the Poor Law Commissioners, 1837–8, 69.
32. Somerville to Henry, 17 October 1832, MH74/12.
33. Somerville to Phillipps, 11 January 1834, *ibid.*
34. Statistics of Students and Subjects, no 2, part 4, MH74/16.
35. Somerville to Hastings, 2 July 1832, MH74/12.
36. Durey, 'Bodysnatchers', 212.
37. Somerville to Sir James Graham, n.d. (1841?), MH74/13.
38. Somerville to Graham, November 1841, *ibid.*
39. Somerville to Phillipps, 13 December 1841, MH74/14.
40. Somerville to Phillipps, 29 March 1842, *ibid*; Durey, 'Bodysnatchers', 224, n.69.
41. Cope, *History of St Mary's Hospital*, 5–7; Holmes, *Brodie*, 111–23.
42. Sheppard, *Local Government in St Marylebone*, 294.
43. Somerville to Grainger, 3 October 1837, MH74/13.
44. Durey, 'Bodysnatchers', 214.
45. Quarterly Report of Inspector of Anatomy, 31 December 1842, MH74/16.
46. Clarke to H.O., 5 December 1833, HO44/26.

47. Somerville to Phillipps, 3 June 1834, MH74/12.
48. *Ibid.*
49. H.O. to Sheffield Lecturers, 19 February 1835, HO83/1; Walton, *Sheffield*, 158; Porter, *Medical School in Sheffield*, 10.
50. Durey, 'Bodysnatchers', 214.

Bibliography

SECTION 1. MANUSCRIPT SOURCES AND COLLECTIONS

A. Public Record Office.

i. Privy Council Papers

PC1/101 PC1/105	Minutes of Central Board of Health, 1831–2
PC1/93 PC1/94 PC1/95	Out-Letters of Central Board of Health, 1831–July 1832
PC1/102 PC1/103 PC1/114	In-Letters to Central Board of Health, 1831–3
PC1/106	Original Foreign Correspondence, 1831
PC1/107	In-Letters from Scotland, December 1831 to May 1832
PC1/108	Correspondence with France: Cholera Returns of Great Britain
PC1/2660 PC1/2662	Quarantine, June 1831 to April 1833
PC1/4395	Miscellaneous, Public Health and Quarantine, 1831–2

ii. Home Office Papers

(*a*) Correspondence and Papers, Domestic and General

HO44/24	Miscellaneous In-Letters, 1831
HO44/25	Miscellaneous In-Letters, 1832
HO44/26	Miscellaneous In-Letters, 1833
HO44/27	Miscellaneous In-Letters, 1834
HO44/30	Miscellaneous In-Letters, 1837
HO44/31	Miscellaneous In-Letters, 1838
HO44/32	Miscellaneous In-Letters, 1839
HO44/49	Miscellaneous In-Letters, 1831–7

(*b*) Police

HO60/2	Magistrates Entry Book, 1831–2
HO61/6	Metropolitan Police Correspondence, January–May 1832

HO62/9	Daily Police Reports, July–December 1832
HO62/10	
HO64/18	Seditious and Libellous Publications

(*c*) Miscellaneous

HO31–17	Minutes of Central Board of Health, 1831–2
HO52/20	Disturbances
HO83/1	Out-Letters, 1832–42, Anatomy Act

iii. Ministry of Health

MH74/12	Out-Letters, Inspector of Anatomy, 1832–5
MH74/13	Letter Book—Anatomy—Miscellaneous, 1835–41
MH74/14	Out-Letters, Inspector of Anatomy, 1841–2
MH74/16	Anatomy Act Statistics, 1842–8
MH74/36	Anatomy Act: Letters and Documents, 1834–90
MH5/1	Minutes of General Board of Health, 1848–9
MH5/2	Minutes of General Board of Health, 1849–50.
MH6/2	Rough Minute Book, General Board of Health, 1848

B. British Museum Additional Manuscripts

Add MS 27791	Place Papers
Add MS 27828	
Add MS 27967	Letters and Documents re Cholera in Norfolk, 1831–2
Add MS 28069	Duke of Leeds' Correspondence, 1831–7
Add MS 39167	Miscellaneous Papers

C. Greater London Record Office

WCS 72	Minutes of Westminster Commission of Sewers
SKCS 61	Minutes of Surrey and Kent Commission of Sewers
THCS 440	Register of the Court of the Tower Hamlets Commission of Sewers
HFCS 25	Minutes of Holborn and Finsbury Commission of Sewers
P71/TMS/514	Minutes of St Thomas Board of Health
P92/SAV/Min	Minutes of St Saviour Southwark Board of Health
P92/CTC/88	Vestry Minutes, Christchurch, Surrey
P82/GEO1/63	St George Bloomsbury, Searcher's Report

D. Guildhall Record Office and Guildhall Library

536 F — Minutes of City of London Board of Health, October 1831—January 1832
536 F — Minutes of City of London Board of Health, January 1832—March 1832
65 F — Minutes of City of London Board of Health, March 1832—September 1834
536 F — City of London Board of Health Committee Papers, November 1831—January 1832
365 F — City of London Board of Health Committee Papers, February—July 1832
365 F — City of London Board of Health Committee Papers, August—September 1832
536 F — City of London Board of Health Letter Book, 1831–3
536 F — Printed Minutes of Court of Common Council, 1831–3
536 F — City of London Board of Health, Accounts, 1831–3
MS 9959 — Portsoken Ward Board of Health Minutes, 1831/2
MS 8305 — Minutes of the Meetings held by the Medical Officers of the Board of Health for the City of London, 1831
MS 2050 — Aldersgate Ward Minute Book, vol 2
MS 779/3 — Vestry Minutes, St Vedast alias Foster, Farringdon Ward
MS 606/2 — Vestry Minutes, St Martin Vintry
MS 1561/1 — Cripplegate Wardmote Minute Book

E. London Public Libraries

i. Westminster

C 971 — Minutes, St George Hanover Square Board of Health, 1831–2
K 405 — Minutes, Liberty of the Rolls Board of Health, 1831–3
G 1009 — Vestry Minutes, St Mary-le-Strand
H 808 — Vestry Minutes, St Clement Danes
H 808 — Vestry Minutes, St Paul Covent Garden

ii. Tower Hamlets

Minutes, St Mary-le-Bow Board of Health
Vestry Minutes, All Saints Poplar
Vestry Minutes, St Matthew Bethnal Green
Vestry Minutes, Christ Church Spitalfields
Vestry Minutes, Holy Trinity Minories
Vestry Minutes, Liberty of Norton Folgate

iii. Tottenham

Minutes, Tottenham Board of Health, 1831–2

iv. Greenwich

Vestry Minutes, Parish of Greenwich

F. Provincial Libraries

i. Manchester

M9/36/1	Proceedings, Manchester Board of Health, November 1831—August 1832
M9/36/2	Proceedings, Manchester Board of Health, August 1832—October 1833
M71/1/2/3	Report, Manchester Cholera Relief Fund Committee, April 1833

ii. Redditch

Minutes, First Board of Health, Tardebigge and Redditch, 1832

iii. York

Acc 108:2	Notebook of George Benson, 1841
Acc 26:4	Select Vestry Minutes, St Lawrence and St Nicholas, York
K 109	Memorials to York Corporation, 1827–1833
M 24	Miscellaneous notices from Board of Health

G. Borthwick Institute of Historical Research, York

PR–HUN 9	Vestry Minutes, Huntington Parish
Y/HTG 14	Vestry Minutes, Holy Trinity Goddramgate
Y/HTM 122	Vestry Minutes, Holy Trinity Micklegate
Y/MG 25	Vestry Minutes, St Martin cum Gregory
Y/MAUR 16	Vestry Minutes, St Maurice
Y/MC 111	Vestry Minutes, St Mary Castlegate
NORT 34	Select Vestry Minutes, Norton

SECTION 2. PARLIAMENTARY AND OFFICIAL REPORTS

Anatomy, Select Committee on, *PP*, 1828, IV.

Doctrine of Contagion in Plague, Select Committee on, *PP*, 1819, II.

Epidemic Cholera of 1848–9, Report of the General Board of Health on, *PP*, 1850, XXI.
Epidemic Cholera in England 1866, Report on, *PP*, 1867–8, XXXVII.
Finance Accounts, House of Commons Sessions Papers, *PP*, 1831–2, XXVI.
Health of Towns, CS on, *PP*, 1840, XI.
Large Towns, First Report of the Commissioners into, *PP*, 1844, XVII.
Large Towns, Second Report of the Commissioners into, *PP*, 1845, XVIII.
Laws relating to Irish and Scottish Vagrants, SC on, *PP*, 1828, IV.
Medical Council, Report from the Treatment Committee of, *PP*, 1854–5, XLV.
Medical Education, SC on, *PP*, 1834, XIII.
Metropolitan Sanitary Commission, First Report of, *PP*, 1847–8, XXXII.
Metropolitan Sewers, SC on, *PP*, 1834, XV.
Metropolitan Water Supplies, SC on, *PP*, 1834, XV.
Metropolitan Water Supply, Reports to the President of the General Board of Health on the, *PP*, 1856, LII.
Metropolitan Workhouses, Report on the Capabilities of, for the Reception and Treatment of Cholera Cases, *PP*, 1847–8, LI.
Poor Law Commissioners, Fourth Annual Report of, *PP*, 1837–8, XXVIII.
Population of Great Britain, Comparative Account of, 1801–31, *PP*, 1831, XVIII.
Quarantine and First Board of Health, Papers on, *PP*, 1831, XVII.
Water to the Metropolis, SC on the supply of, *PP*, 1828, VIII.

SECTION 3. PRINTED PRIMARY SOURCES

Hansard.
London Gazette
Local Reports on the Sanitary Condition of the Labouring Population of Great Britain, 1842.
Reports on the Sanitary Condition of the Labouring Population of Scotland, 1842.

SECTION 4. CONTEMPORARY NEWSPAPERS

Aris's Birmingham Gazette
Bristol Mercury

Bristol Mirror
Cobbett's Weekly Political Register
Cornubian
Cosmopolite
Devil in London
Examiner
Figaro in London
Hull Portfolio
Leeds Intelligencer
Leeds Mercury
Liverpool Chronicle
Liverpool Courier
Morning Chronicle
Morning Post
Newcastle Chronicle
Newcastle Courant
North Briton
Nottingham Journal and General Advertiser
Plymouth, Devonport and Stonehouse Herald
Poor Man's Advocate
Poor Man's Guardian
Republican
Republican and Radical Reformer
Royal Cornwall Gazette
Sheffield Independent
Sheffield Mercury
Stafford County Herald
Staffordshire Advertiser
Staffordshire Gazette
Sunderland Herald
Times
True Sun
West Briton
Wolverhampton Chronicle
York Courant
York Herald
Yorkshire Gazette

SECTION 5. CONTEMPORARY JOURNALS AND PERIODICALS

Annual Register
Blackwood's Magazine

Cholera Gazette
Edinburgh Medical and Surgical Journal
Gentlemen's Magazine
Journal of the London Statistical Society
Lancet
London Medical Gazette
London Medical and Physical Journal
London Medical and Surgical Journal
Medico-Chirurgical Review
Quarterly Review
Tait's Edinburgh Magazine
Transactions of the Provincial Medical and Surgical Association

SECTION 6. CONTEMPORARY AUTHORITIES

(The place of publication is London unless otherwise stated.)

Alderson, J., *A Brief Outline of the History and Progress of Cholera at Hull with some Remarks on the Pathology and Treatment of the Disease*, 1832.

Anderson, W. S., 'An Account of the Cholera Morbus Epidemic in India in 1817', *EMSJ*, xv, 1819.

Anon, *An Enquiry into the Remote Causes of Cholera*, Edinburgh 1832.

Anon, *Why Are You Afraid of the Cholera?, and the Sure Remedy*, 1832.

Armstrong, H. K. & Edgar, S., *Observations on Malignant Cholera, as it Occurred at Prestonpans, Cockenzie and Portseton*, Edinburgh 1832.

Baines, E., *History, Directory, Gazetteer* (sic) *of the County Palatine of Lancaster*, 2 vols, Liverpool 1825.

Baines, T., *History of the Commerce and Town of Liverpool*, 1852.

Baker, R., *Report of the Leeds Board of Health*, Leeds 1833.

Barry, D., *Experimental Researches, on the Influence Exerted by Atmospheric Pressure on the Progression of the Blood in the Veins*, 1826.

Barry, D., 'Remarks on the Gibraltar Epidemic', i, *LMPJ*, new series x, 1831.

Barry, D., 'Remarks on the Gibraltar Epidemic', ii, *LMPJ*, new series, xi, 1831.

Barry, D., 'On the Statistics of Cholera,' *JLSS*, i, 1837.

Bell, G. H., *Treatise on Cholera Asphyxia*, London and Edinburgh 1831, 2nd ed. 1832.

Boyle, J., *A Treatise on the Cholera Epidemic in India*, 1821.

Burdekin, R., *An Historical Account of the Plague and Other Pestilential Disorders... and an Account of the Cholera Morbus*, York 1832.

Carrick, A. & Symonds, A., 'Medical Topography of Bristol', *TPMSA*, ii, 1834.

Chadwick, E., *Report on the Sanitary Condition of the Labouring Population in Great Britain, 1842*, 1842, new ed., Edinburgh 1965.

Chadwick, E., *Supplementary Report on the Practice of Interment in Towns*, 1843.

Christison, R., 'Account of the Arrangements made by the Edinburgh Board of Health, Preparatory to the Arrival of Cholera in that City', *EMSJ*, xxxvii, 1832.

Clanny, W. R., *Hyperanthraxis: or the Cholera in Sunderland*, 1832.

Coppard, Rev. W. I., *Cottage Scenes During the Cholera*, 1848.

Corbyn, F., *A Treatise on the Epidemic Cholera as it has Prevailed in India*, Calcutta 1832.

Craigie, D., 'Account of the Epidemic Cholera of Newburn', *EMSJ*, xxxvii, 1832.

Davis, T., *Sewage or Drainage, considered in Connexion with Cholera and the General Health and Improvement of the Metropolis*, 1832.

Engels, F., *The Condition of the Working Class in England in 1844*, 1892, reprinted in Edinburgh 1968.

Forster, T., *Essay on the Origins, Symptoms and Treatment of Cholera Morbus*, 1831.

French, J. G., *A Letter Addressed to the Central Board of Health*, 1832.

Gaskell, S., 'Cholera in Manchester', *EMSJ*, xl, 1833.

Gaulter, H., *The Origins and Progress of the Malignant Cholera in Manchester*, 1833.

George, H., *Practical Observations on Cholera*, 1834.

Girdlestone, Rev. C., *Seven Sermons Preached during the Prevalence of Cholera, in the Parish of Sedgeley*, 1833.

Greenhow, E. H., 'Cholera in Tynemouth in 1831–2, 1848–9, and 1853', *Transactions of the Epidemiological Society of London*, 1855.

Greenhow, T. M., *Cholera, as it has recently Appeared in the Towns of Newcastle and Gateshead*, 1832.

Haslewood, W. & Mordey, W., *History and Medical Treatment of Cholera in Sunderland*, 1832.

Hodgkin, T., *Hints Relating to the Cholera in London*, 1832.

Kay, J. P., *The Moral and Physical Condition of the Working Classes Employed in the Cotton Manufacture of Manchester*, 2nd ed. 1832, reprinted 1970.

Kell, J. B., *On The Appearance of Cholera at Sunderland in 1831*, Edinburgh 1834.

Kendrick, J., *Cursory Remarks on the Present Epidemic*, 1832.

Kennedy, J., *The History of the Contagious Cholera*, 1831.

Lawrie, J. A., *Essay on the Cholera in India, and in Sunderland, Newcastle and Gateshead*, Glasgow 1832.

Laycock, T., *Report on the State of York*, York 1843.

Leigh, Rev. W., *An Authentic Narrative of the Melancholy Occurrences at Bilston in the County of Stafford, during the Awful Visitation in that Town by Cholera in the months of August and September 1832*, Wolverhampton 1833.

Lizars, J., *Substance of the Investigations regarding Cholera Asphyxia*, Edinburgh 1832.

Macmichael, W., *Is the Cholera Spasmodica of India a Contagious Disease?*, 1831.

Molison, T., *Remarks on the Epidemic Disease called Cholera, as it occurred in Newcastle*, 2nd ed. Edinburgh 1832.

Monk, W., *Roll of the Royal College of Physicians*, Vol. 3, 1878.

Needham, J. P., *Facts and Observations on the Cholera in York*, York 1832.

Ogier Ward, T., 'Observations upon Cholera, as it appeared in Wolverhampton and its Neighbourhood in August, September and October 1832', *TPMSA*, ii, 1834.

Orton, R., *An Essay on the Epidemic Cholera in India*, 2nd ed. 1831.

O'Shaughnessy, W. B., 'Proposal of a New Method of Treating the Blue Epidemic Cholera by the Injection of Highly-oxygenised Salts into the Venous System', *The Lancet*, i, 1831–2.

O'Shaughnessy, W. B., *Report of the Chemical Pathology of the Malignant Cholera*, 1832.

Pettigrew, T. J., *Biographical Memoirs of the Most Celebrated Physicians and Surgeons*, 1838.

Searle, C., *Cholera, Its Nature, Cause, Treatment and Prevention*, 1831.

Shapter, T., *The History of the Cholera in Exeter in 1832*, 1849.

Somerville, J. C., *A Letter Addressed to the Lord Chancellor on the Study of Anatomy*, 1832.

Stevens, W. B., 'On the Efficiency of Saline Agents in the Treatment of West Indian Fevers', *The Lancet*, i, 1831–2.

Smith, J., *Report of the State of the City of York and Other Towns*, 1845.

Streeten, R., 'Report on the State of Disease in the City of Worcester, during the year 1832, *TPMSA*, i, 1833.
Symonds, J. A., 'Remarks upon the Progress and Causes of Cholera, as it occurred in Bristol, in 1832', *TPMSA*, iii, 1834.
Thackrah, C. T., *The Effects of Arts, Trades and Professions on Health and Longevity*, 1831, reprinted Edinburgh 1957.
Thackrah, C. T., *Cholera: Its Character and Treatment*, Leeds 1832.
Walker, G., *Gatherings from Graveyards*, 1839.
Winterbottom, T. M., 'Thoughts on Quarantine and Contagion', *EMSJ*, xxx, 1828.

SECTION 7. MODERN SECONDARY SOURCES

(a) Books and Monographs

Ackerknecht, E. H., *A Short History of Medicine*, New York 1968.
Allport, G. & Postman, L., *The Psychology of Rumour*, New York 1948.
Altick, R. D., *Victorian Studies in Scarlet*, 1973.
Andrews, W. (ed.), *The Doctor in History, Literature, Folk-lore*, Hull 1896.
Apsinall, A. (ed.), *Three Early Nineteenth-Century Diaries*, 1952.
Badham, P., *Christian Beliefs About Life and Death*, 1976.
Baker, G. & Chapman, D. (eds), *Man and Society in Disaster*, New York, 1962.
Bailey, J. B. (ed.), *The Diary of a Resurrectionist, 1811–12*, 1896.
Ball, J. M., *The Sack-Em-Up Men*, 1928.
Barton, N., *The Lost Rivers of London*, 1965.
Bickerton, T. H., *A Medical History of Liverpool from the Earliest Days to the Year 1920*, 1936.
Biraben, J-N., *Les Hommes et la Peste*, Paris 1976.
Branch Johnson, W., *The English Prison Hulks*, Sussex 1970.
Briggs, A., *Victorian Cities*, 1963.
Briggs A. & Savile, J. (eds), *Essays in Labour History*, 1967.
Brockington, C. F., *Public Health in the Nineteenth Century*, Edinburgh 1965.
Brook, C., *Battling Surgeon*, Glasgow 1945.
Buchanan, G., *On the Effects of the Anatomy Act, and the Facilities for the Study of Practical Anatomy in Glasgow*, Glasgow 1860?
Buer, M. C., *Health, Wealth and Population in the Early Days of the Industrial Revolution*, 1926.
Burnett, J., *Plenty and Want*, 1966.

Butler, J. R. M., *The Passing of the Great Reform Bill*, 1914, reprinted 1963.

Carnall, R., *Robert Southey and His Age*, 1960.

Chandler, G., *Liverpool*, 1957.

Chevalier, L. (ed.), *Le Choléra, La Première Épidémie du xixe Siècle*, La Roche-sur-Yon 1958.

Chevalier, L., *Labouring Classes and Dangerous Classes in Paris in the First Half of the Nineteenth Century*, 1973.

Cipolla, C., *Cristofano and The Plague*, 1973.

Clark, Sir G., *A History of the Royal College of Physicians*, 2 vols, 1966.

Clark, G. Kitson, *Churchmen and the Condition of England, 1832–85*, 1973.

Cole, H., *Things for the Surgeons, A History of the Body Snatchers*, 1964.

Coleman, B. I. (ed.), *The Idea of the City in Nineteenth-Century Britain*, 1973.

Cordell, A., *The Fire People*, 1973.

Creighton, C., *History of Epidemics in Britain*, 2 vols, 1894, reprinted 1965.

Crosse, V. M., *A Surgeon in the Early Nineteenth Century*, 1968.

Dent, R., *The Making of Birmingham*, Birmingham 1894.

Durey, M., *The First Spasmodic Cholera Epidemic in York, 1832*, York 1974.

Dyos, H. J. (ed.), *Victorian Suburb, A Study of the Growth of Camberwell*, Leicester 1966.

Dyos, H. J. & Wolff, M. (eds), *The Victorian City, Images and Realities*, 2 vols, 1973.

Farr, W., *Vital Statistics*, 1885.

Finer, S. E., *The Life and Times of Sir Edwin Chadwick*, 1952.

Foster, J., *Class Struggle and the Industrial Revolution*, 1974.

Frazer, W. M., *A History of English Public Health, 1834–1939*, 1950.

Gale, A. H., *Epidemic Diseases*, 1959.

Gauldie, E., *Cruel Habitations: A History of Working Class Housing, 1780–1918*, 1974

George, D., *London Life in the Eighteenth Century*, 1925.

Goodman, L. S. & Gilman, A., *The Pharmacological Basis of Therapeutics*, 3rd ed. New York 1966.

Hamburger, J., *Intellectuals in Politics, John Stuart Mill and the Philosophic Radicals*, Yale 1965.

Hamburger, J., *James Mill and the Art of Revolution*, 1963.

Hamilton-Jenkins, A. K., *Cornwall and Its People*, Newton Abbot 1970.

Hammond, J. L. & B., *The Skilled Labourer*, New York 1970.
Hammond, J. L. & B., *The Town Labourer*, New York 1968.
Henderson, W., *Folk Lore of the Northern Counties of England and the Borders*, 1866, reprinted Wakefield 1973.
Hill, A., *Seventy Two Years in Tottenham*, 1899.
Hobsbawm, E. & Rudé, G., *Captain Swing*, 1970.
Hobson, W., *World Health and History*, Bristol 1963.
Hole, C., *English Folklore*, 1940.
Hollaender, A. E. J. & Kellaway, W. (eds), *Studies in London History*, 1969.
Hollis, P., *The Pauper Press*, 1970.
Holmes, R., *That Alarming Malady: An Account of the Cholera Epidemic in Ely*, 1832, Ely 1974.
Inglis, B., *Poverty and the Industrial Revolution*, 1971.
Jephson, H., *The Sanitary Evolution of London*, 1907.
Jewitt, L., *A History of Plymouth*, 1873.
Jones, D. J. V., *Before Rebecca: Popular Protest in Wales, 1793–1835*, 1973.
Jordan, F. W., *The Life of Joseph Jordan, Surgeon*, Manchester 1904.
Keele, K., *The Evolution of Clinical Methods in Medicine*, 1963.
Kendall, H., *The Origins of the Primitive Methodist Church*, 2 vols, 1905.
Kirkman Gray, B., *A History of English Philanthropy*, 1905, reprinted 1967.
Kuhn, T., *The Structure of Scientific Revolutions*, 1970.
Lambert, R., *Sir John Simon and English Social Administration*, 1963.
Langdon-Brown, Sir W., *Some Chapters in Cambridge Medical History*, Cambridge 1946.
Langford, J. A., *A Century of Birmingham Life*, 2 vols, Birmingham 1868.
Latimer, J., *The Annals of Bristol in the Nineteenth Century*, Bristol 1887.
Lefebvre, G., *The Great Fear of 1789. Rural Panic In Revolutionary France*, 1973.
Lewis, O., *A Death in the Sanchez Family*, 1969.
Lewis, R. A., *Edwin Chadwick and the Public Health Movement*, 1952.
Lifton, R. J., *Death in Life: Survivors of Hiroshima*, New York 1967.
Lifton, R. J. & Olson, R., *Explorations in Psychohistory: The Wellfleet Papers*, 1974.
Londonderry, Edith Marchioness of, *Frances Anne. The Life and*

Times of Frances Anne, Marchioness of Londonderry and her husband Charles, 1958.
Longmate, N., *King Cholera. The Biography of a Disease*, 1966.
Lovett, W., *Life and Struggles of William Lovett*, 1876, reprinted 1967.
Macmichael, W. & Munk, W., *The Gold Headed Cane*, 1884.
Macnamara, N. C., *Asiatic Cholera: Its History up to 15 July 1892, Causes and Treatment*, 1892.
Malinowski, B., *Magic, Science and Religion and Other Essays*, New York, 1954.
Mathias, P. (ed.), *Science and Society, 1600–1900*, Cambridge 1972.
McGrew, R., *Russia and the Cholera 1823–32*, Wisconsin 1965.
McGrigor, Sir J., *The Autobiography and Services of Sir James McGrigor, Bart*, 1861.
Muir, R., *A History of Liverpool*, 1907.
Owen, D., *English Philanthropy, 1660–1960*, 1965.
Peet, H. (ed.), *Liverpool Vestry Books, 1681–1834*, 1915.
Pelling, M., *Cholera, Fever and English Medicine*, Oxford 1978.
Pollitzer, R., *Cholera*, Geneva 1959.
Porter, W. S., *The Medical School in Sheffield, 1828–1928*, Sheffield 1928.
Poynter, F. N. L. (ed.), *Medicine and Science in the 1860s*, 1968.
Poynter, J. R., *Society and Pauperism: English Ideas on Poor Relief, 1795–1834*, 1969.
Radzinowicz, L., *A History of English Criminal Law and Its Administration from 1750*, iv, 1968.
Razzell, P. & Wainwright, R. (eds), *The Victorian Working Class*, 1973.
Redford, A., *Labour Migration in England, 1800–50*, 1926.
Reeve, H. (ed.), *The Greville Memoirs*, 1888.
Roberts, D., *Victorian Origins of the British Welfare State*, Yale 1960.
Robson, B. T., *Urban Growth: An Approach*, 1973.
Rosenberg, C., *The Cholera Years. The United States in 1832, 1849 and 1866*, Chicago 1962.
Rudé, G., *Hanoverian London, 1714–1808*, 1971.
Rudé, G., *Paris and London in the Eighteenth Century*, 1970.
Sand, R., *The Advance to Social Medicine*, 1952.
Sanger, 'Lord' G., *Seventy Years a Showman*, reprinted 1966.
Scott, Sir H. H., *Some Notable Epidemics*, 1934.
Sheppard, F. H. W., *Local Government in St. Marylebone, 1688–1835*, 1958.

Sheppard, F. H. W., *London 1808–70: The Infernal Wen*, 1971.
Shibutani, T. (ed.), *Human Nature and Collective Behaviour*, Prentice Hall 1970.
Shyrock, R. H., *The Development of Modern Medicine*, 1948.
Siegfried, A., *Germs and Ideas*, Edinburgh 1965.
Sigerist, H. E., *Civilisation and Disease*, 2nd ed. 1965.
Singer, C., *A Short History of Medicine*, 1944.
Smelser, N. J., *Theory of Collective Behaviour*, 1962.
Smiles, A., *Samuel Smiles and His Surroundings*, 1956.
Snow, J., *Snow on Cholera. Being a Reprint of Two Papers*, New York and London 1965.
Sprigge, S., *The Life and Times of Thomas Wakley*, 1899.
Steiner, I. D. & Fishbein, M. (eds), *Current Studies in Social Psychology*, New York 1966.
Stevens, W. R., *Life and Letters of Dean Hook*, 2 vols. Bentley 1878.
Stokes, J., *History of the Epidemic Cholera in Sheffield in 1832*, Sheffield 1921.
Stranks, C. J., *Dean Hook*, 1954.
Sutherland, C. (ed.), *Studies in the Growth of Nineteenth Century Government*, 1972.
Sykes, L. & K., *Sketches of the Life of Edward Jackson of Leeds*, 1912.
Taylor, A. J., *Laissez Faire and State Intervention in Nineteenth Century Britain*, 1972.
Taylor, A. J. (ed.), *The Standard of Living in Britain in the Industrial Revolution*, 1975.
Thale, M. (ed.), *The Autobiography of Francis Place*, Cambridge 1972.
Tholfsen, T., *Working Class Radicalism in Mid-Victorian England*, 1976.
Thompson, E. P., *The Making of the English Working Class*, 1963.
Thompson, E. P. & Yeo, E. (eds), *The Unknown Mayhew, Selections from the Morning Chronicle 1849–50*, 1973.
Top, F. H. & Wehrle, P. H. (eds), *Communicable and Infectious Diseases*, 8th ed., St Louis 1976.
Toynbee, A. J. *et al.*, *Man's Concern with Death*, 1968.
Turner, C. H., *The Inhumanists*, 1932.
Underwood, E. A. (ed.), *Science, Medicine and History: Essays in Honour of Charles Singer*, 2 vols, 1953.
Wallas, G., *The Life of Francis Place*, 1925.
Walton, M., *Sheffield: Its Story and Achievements*, Sheffield 1948.
Ward, J. T. (ed.), *Popular Movements, c. 1830–50*, 1970.
Ward, J. T., *The Factory System*, 2 vols, Newton Abbott 1970.

Wearmouth, R. F., *Some Working Class Movements of the Nineteenth Century*, 1948.
Webb, S. & B., *English Local Government: Statutory Authorities for Special Purposes*, 1922.
Weiner, J., *The War of the Unstamped*, Ithaca 1969.
Williams, G. A., *The Merthyr Rising*, 1978.
Winslow, C. E. A., *The Conquest of Epidemic Disease*, Princeton 1943.
Woodhead, T. W., *History of the Huddersfield Water Supplies*, Huddersfield 1939.
Woodward, J., *To Do The Sick No Harm*, 1974.
Woodward, J. & Richards, D. (eds), *Health Care and Popular Medicine in Nineteenth-Century England*, 1976.
Woodward, Sir L., *The Age of Reform*, 1962.
Zacke, B., *Kolera Epidemien i Stockholm 1834*, Stockholm 1971.

(b) Articles and Essays

Ackerknecht, E. H., 'Anti-contagionism between 1827 and 1867', *BHM*, xxviii, 1948.
Baehrel, R., 'Épidémie et Terreur : histoire et sociologie', *Annales Historiques de la Révolution Française*, xxiii, 1951.
Baehrel, R., 'La haine de classe en temps d'épidémie', *Annales ESC*, vii, 1952.
Banerjea, A. C., 'Note on Cholera in the United Provinces (Uttar Pradesh)', *Indian Journal of Medical Research*, xxxix, 1951.
Bell, J. H., 'Some Fragments of Local Medical History', *Bradford Antiquary*, i, 1888.
Benenson, A. S., 'Cholera', *Communicable and Infectious Diseases*, eds Top & Wehrle.
Bonser, K. J., 'Spas, Wells and Springs of Leeds', *Publications of the Thoresby Society (Miscellany)*, xvi, 1974.
Briggs, A., 'Cholera and Society in the Nineteenth Century', *P & P*, xix, 1961.
Briggs, A., 'The Language of "Class" in Early Nineteenth-Century England', *Essays in Labour History*, eds Briggs & Savile.
Brockington, C. F., 'Public Health at the Privy Council, 1831–4', *JHM*, xvi, 1961.
Chapman, D. W., 'A Brief Introduction to Contemporary Disaster Research', *Man and Society in Disaster*, eds Baker & Chapman.
Durey, M. J., 'Bodysnatchers and Benthamites : the implications of the Dead Body Bill for the London Schools of Anatomy, 1820–42', *The London Journal*, ii, 1976.
Eckman, J., 'Anglo-Amercan Hostility in American Medical Literature of the Nineteenth Century', *BHM*, ix, 1941.

Eversley, D., 'Le Choléra en Angleterre', *Le Choléra*, ed. Chevalier.
Eyler, J. M., 'William Farr on the Cholera : the sanitarians' disease theory and the statisticians' method', *JHM*, xxviii, 1973.
Finer, S. E., 'The Transmission of Benthamite Ideas, 1820–50', *Studies in the Growth of Nineteenth Century Government*, ed. Sutherland.
Fleetwood, J. M., 'The Irish Resurrectionists', *Irish Journal of Medical Science*, 1959.
Fraser, D., 'The Movement for Reform', *Popular Movements*, ed. Ward.
Frieden, N., 'The Russian Cholera Epidemic, 1892–93, and Medical Professionalisation', *JSH*, x, 1977.
Greenwood, M., 'Miasma and Contagion', *Science, Medicine and History*, ed. Underwood.
Greig, E. D. W., 'The Treatment of Cholera by Intravenous Saline Injections', *Edinburgh Medical Journal*, liii, 1946.
Gutchen, R. M., 'Local Improvements and Centralisation in Nineteenth-Century England', *HJ*, iv, 1961.
Hennock, E. P., 'Urban Sanitary Reform a Generation Before Chadwick?', *EcHR*, 2nd series, x, 1957.
Hewitt, G., 'Cholera in Beith, 1832–4', *Ayrshire Archaeological and Natural History Collections*, 2nd series, viii, 1969.
Holloway, S. W. F., 'The Apothecaries' Act 1815 : A Reinterpretation', *M.H.*, x, 1966.
Howard-Jones, N., 'Cholera Therapy in the Nineteenth Century', *JHM*, xxviii, 1972.
Inkster, I., 'Marginal Men : aspects of the social role of the medical community in Sheffield, 1790–1850', *Health Care and Popular Medicine*, eds Woodward & Richards.
Jones, G. P., 'The Cholera in Wales', *National Library of Wales Journal*, x, 1957–8.
Keith-Lucas, B., 'Some Influences Affecting the Development of Sanitary Legislation in England', *EcHR*, 2nd series, vi, 1954.
Kerckhoff. A. C., 'A Theory of Hysterical Contagion', *Human Nature*, ed. Shibutani.
King, L.S., 'The Blood-letting Controversy : a study of the scientific method', *BHM*, xxxv, 1961.
Lampard, E. E., 'The Urbanising World', *The Victorian City*, eds Dyos & Wolff.
Langtry, D. A., 'The 1832 Epidemic of Asiatic Cholera in New Haven, Connecticut', *JHM*, xxv, 1970.
Law, C. M., 'The Growth of Urban Population in England and Wales, 1801–1911', *Transactions of the Institute of British Geographers*, xli, 1967.

Lifton, R. J., 'The Sense of Immortality: On Death and the Continuity of Life', *Explorations in Psychohistory*, eds Lifton & Olson.

Luckin, W., 'The Final Catastrophe—Cholera in London 1866', *MH*, xxi, 1977.

Macdonagh, O., 'The Nineteenth-Century Revolution in Government', *HJ*, i, 1958.

McDonald, J. C., 'The History of Quarantine in Britain during the nineteenth century', *BHM*, xxv, 1951.

McGrew, R. E., 'The First Cholera Epidemic and Social History', *BHM*, xxxiv, 1960.

McKeown, T., 'A Sociological Approach to the History of Medicine', *MH*, xiv, 1970.

Mitchell, G., 'Anatomical and Resurrectionist Activities in North Scotland', *JHM*, iv, 1959.

Morris, R. J., 'Religion and Medicine: the Cholera pamphlets of Oxford, 1832, 1849 and 1854', *MH*, xix, 1975.

Niebyl, P. H., 'The English Bloodletting Revolution, or Modern Medicine before 1850', *BHM*, li, 1977.

Oram, R. B., 'Old London Bridge', *History Today*, vi, 1956.

Parris, H., 'The Nineteenth-Century Revolution in Government: a Reappraisal Reappraised', *HJ*, ii, 1960.

Peacock, A. J., 'York and the Resurrection Men', *York History*, i, 1974?

Power, D., 'The Medical Institutions of London', *British Medical Journal*, ii, 1895.

Price-Williams, R., 'The Population of London, 1801–81', *JRSS*, xlviii, 1885.

Prothero, I., 'William Benbow and the Concept of the General Strike', *P & P*, lxiii, 1974.

Roberts, F., 'The Effects of Epidemics on Population and Social Life', *Proceedings of the Royal Society of Medicine*, 1955.

Rollet, C. & Souriac, A., 'Le Choléra de 1832 en Seine et Oise', *Annales ESC*, xxix, 1974.

Rosen, G., 'Cameralism and the Concept of a Medical Police', *BHM*, xxvii, 1953.

Rosen, G., 'C. T. Thackrah in the Agitation for Factory Reform', *British Journal of Industrial Medicine*, x, 1953.

Rosen, G., 'Disease and Social Criticism: a contribution to the theory of medical history', *BHM*, x, 1941.

Rosen, G., 'People, Disease and Emotion: some newer problems for research in medical history', *BHM*, xli, 1967.

Rosen, G., 'Disease, Debility and Death', *The Victorian City*, eds Dyos & Wolff, vol 2.

Rosenberg, C., 'Cholera in Nineteenth-Century Europe; a tool for social and economic analysis', *Comparative Studies in Society and History*, 1965–6.
Rosenberg, C., 'The Cause of Cholera: aspects of etiological thought in nineteenth-century America', *BHM*, xxxiv, 1960.
Rowe, D. J., 'Class and Political Radicalism in London, 1831–2', *HJ*, xiii, 1970.
Rowe, D. J., 'Francis Place and the Historian', *HJ*, xvi, 1973.
Rudé, G., 'English Rural and Urban Disturbances on the Eve of the First Reform Bill, 1830–1', *P & P*, xxxvii, 1967.
Samuel, R., 'Comers and Goers', *The Victorian City*, eds Dyos & Wolff, Vol. 1.
Sarnoff, I. & Zimbardo, P. G., 'Anxiety, Fear and Social Affiliation', *Current Studies in Social Psychology*, eds Steiner & Fishbein.
Shannon, H. A., 'Migration and the Growth of London, 1841–91', *EcHR*, 1st series, i, 1935.
Sigsworth, E., 'Gateways to Death? Medicine, Hospitals and Mortality, 1700–1850', *Science and Society, 1600–1900*, ed. Mathias.
Thomas, W. E. S., 'James Mill's Politics: the "Essay on Government" and the movement for Reform', *HJ*, xii, 1969.
Thompson, E. P., 'The Moral Economy of the Crowd', *P & P*, L, 1971.
Underwood, E. A., 'The History of Cholera in Great Britain', *Proceedings of the Royal Society of Medicine*, 1948.
Underwood, E. A., 'The History of the 1832 Cholera Epidemic in Yorkshire', *Proceedings of the Royal Society of Medicine*, 1934–5.
Waddington, I., 'General Practitioners and Consultants in Early Nineteenth-Century England: the Sociology of an Intra-Professional Conflict', *Health Care and Popular Medicine*, eds Woodward & Richards.

(c) Theses

Fielder, G. D., Public Health and Hospital Administration in Nineteenth-Century Swansea, M.A. thesis, University of Swansea 1962.
Gatherer, A., A Socio-Medical Study of the First Cholera Epidemic in Great Britain, D.M. thesis, University of Aberdeen, 1960.
Morris, R. J., The Organisation and Aims of the Principal Secular Voluntary Organisations of the Leeds Middle Class 1830–51, D.Phil. thesis, University of Oxford 1971.

Index